Advanced Praise

"Explaining what goes on in our brain and body when we are stressed is not an easy task. Dr. Ramos does an excellent job by also explaining what we can do about it in steps that we all can take."

Bruce S. McEwen, Ph.D.
Alfred E. Mirsky Professor of Neuroendocrinology and
Stress at The Rockefeller University and author of
The End of Stress As We Know It *and* The Hostage Brain

"As a professional athlete, I can relate to a life full of stress, pressure, and expectations. In this book, Dr. Ramos takes the time to explain what stress really is and provides strategies to help relax your mind and minimize stress in your life. I really enjoyed his natural solutions to deal with stress, focusing on nutrition, meditation, body awareness, etc.

I have had the chance to work with nutritionist, trainers and therapist throughout my career to take care of my body and physical health, but the mind is a whole different story. I have dealt with insomnia and extreme fatigue due to stress and pressure.

This book has helped me focus on the mind side of it all. Dr. Ramos offers strategies and an easy meditation program to help you be aware and focus on yourself to better relax and recover. I have just pointed out a part of the book that really had an impact in my journey, but Dr. Ramos offers a bigger picture with many more strategies that can impact many people with different needs."

Xavier Ouellet
Professional Defenseman of the National
Hockey League, Montreal Canadiens

"What an extraordinary book Dr. Ramos has written! To say that he put his heart and soul into this is an understatement! With all his heart he is committed to your health and happiness. In this book it is impossible to miss Dr. Ramos' commitment to his clients and his dedication to what he has studied, learned, and applied as the path for his clients' wellness, body, mind, heart, and spirit.

This is a masterful book! If you have any issues with stress ~ and who does not! ~ check this book out. His work is comprehensive and powerful, a definite must read for anyone suffering from symptoms linked to stress and anxiety. Thank you, Brian, for your brilliant addition to the 'healthy and happy' conversation!"

Reverend Katherine McClelland
Minister, Speaker, Spiritual-Life Coach, and Author of
Breathless: The Relentless Pursuit of the Good Life

The Art of Stress-Free Living

The ART *of* STRESS-FREE LIVING

Reprogram
Your Life
From the
Inside Out

Brian P. Ramos, PH.D.

NEW YORK

LONDON • NASHVILLE • MELBOURNE • VANCOUVER

The Art of Stress-Free Living
Reprogram Your Life From the Inside Out

Published in New York, New York, by Morgan James Publishing in partnership with Difference Press. Morgan James is a trademark of Morgan James, LLC. www.MorganJamesPublishing.com

ISBN 9781642795806 paperback
ISBN 9781642795813 eBook
Library of Congress Control Number: 2019939446

Cover Design by:
Alexander Canino

Interior Design by:
Christopher Kirk
www.GFSstudio.com

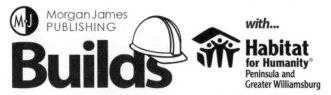

Morgan James is a proud partner of Habitat for Humanity Peninsula and Greater Williamsburg. Partners in building since 2006.

Get involved today! Visit
MorganJamesPublishing.com/giving-back

*To my wife Norma, for always being there
and giving her all even when faced with adversity.*

Table of Contents

Foreword

S tress is everywhere in our fast-paced, pressured lives, often leaving us frazzled and feeling out of control. Dr. Ramos' new book, *The Art of Stress-Free Living*, teaches us about how stress alters our bodies and brains, and offers coping strategies to regain our sense of efficacy and joy in our lives.

Dr. Ramos performed his doctoral thesis in my lab at Yale University, exploring how stress and age can impair our prefrontal cortex, a newly evolved brain region that subserves higher cognition. The prefrontal cortex sits behind our foreheads in the front of the brain and is responsible for a remarkable set of higher cognitive abilities, including abstract thought, higher reasoning, and the generation of language.

The prefrontal cortex also provides the so-called executive functions that apply "top-down" control over our actions, thoughts, and emotions. It helps us screen out distractions and organize for the future and give us insight about others and ourselves. There is also evidence that the prefrontal cortex is lateralized in humans, with the right hemisphere being specialized for inhibiting inappropriate actions, thoughts, and emotions, while the left hemisphere generates language and can serve as a sort of "mental cheerleader."

Exposure to stress can rapidly take the prefrontal cortex "off-line," especially when we feel we have no control over the stressor. At the same time, stress strengthens more primitive parts of the brain such as the amygdala and the striatum that mediate unconscious emotional responses and habits. In this way, we rapidly switch from a reflective to a reflexive state. This may save our life in some situations, e.g., when we are cut off on the highway while driving or when we are in danger and need to be distracted by small changes in the environment. However, losing prefrontal function can be very harmful when we are in situations that require high order function, e.g. taking an important exam or listening to a doctor's instructions. Unfortunately, these brain changes can be exaggerated with chronic stress exposure, when we lose prefrontal gray matter while primitive brain circuits can grow stronger, engraining unhealthy responses.

Luckily, the effects of stress on the brain can be reversed. In some situations, we can learn to gain a sense of control over the situation, or if that is not possible, we can learn to do things that can reduce our body and brain's response to the stress. For example, deep breathing has been shown to quiet one of the brain's stress centers, the locus coeruleus in the brainstem, and helps to calm behavior in mice.

In this book, Dr. Ramos provides many strategies to help you learn to better cope with stress. He has a rare, multi-faceted view on stress: he has a Ph.D. in neuroscience, but also has a master yoga practice, including advanced experience with meditation, concentration, Ayurveda, mindfulness, and breathing techniques.

Dr. Ramos dispels the notion that stress is our enemy, and instead describes lifestyle changes and techniques that he has used and perfected that can help make stress your ally. He describes the lessons he has learned from these very different worlds that can help to give perspective and a healthier response to stress exposure. And he reminds us that both the ancient wisdom of the Vedas and the newer wisdom of neuroscience tell us that it is how we perceive a stressor that determines whether it defeats us or brings us to a deeper level of understanding.

> "Light finds her treasure of colours
> through the antagonism of clouds."
> — Rabindranath Tagore, *Fireflies*

Amy F.T. Arnsten, Ph.D.
Bethany, CT

Introduction:

This Book Is for You

"Synchronicity is an ever-present reality
for those who have the eyes to see."

— Carl Jung

I write this book for you from the heart to transform your relationship with your body, mind, and spirit in a way that will allow you to become more patient and accepting of yourself. I write this as a friend who has seen what stress can do to a loved one. I want for you to find the comfort and peace that you deserve. I hope that what I am ready to share with the world will be of value to you.

This book is a practical guide, of sorts, to help you begin a journey of self-discovery. May you transcend lower levels of self and move into higher realms where you can enjoy greater happiness, tranquility, and health with your partner and loved ones. Within are a series of tools and a process that I wish to share with you in the hopes that we can connect in whichever way is most helpful to you throughout this journey.

I do not want to see you walling yourself up or anesthetizing yourself to avoid life's stresses, for attempting to escape or avoid your problems will only bring you and your loved ones more pain and conflict. You deserve to be free and joyous in the present, and together I know that we can figure out how to face your problems and stressors head on.

I have dedicated more than two decades to mastering the art of conscious living, and I wish to share some of the secrets I have learned with you to inspire you to reach new heights as part of a self-directed self-care program tailor-made to your constitution, personality, body type, age, etc. To do this, I will make myself available to work with you as my client, if you wish, to provide a different way to approach health and well-being by caring for the multidimensional and unique person that you are. Programs that offer blanket solutions may work to some extent, but just like our current pharmacologically-driven medical system, it does not come without its shortcomings and even side effects.

This book will help to teach you the art of mastering life by bringing you into a state that you may have long forgotten. The goal, in many ways, is to help reconnect you with your inner child full of playfulness, laughter, and joy, even in the most hectic of circumstances. You can certainly learn to open your heart like a child to discover bliss and contentment without sacrificing success in worldly or business matters.

Indeed, you can learn to be successful in life and have a high-powered career without sacrificing your happiness, health, or peace of mind. Why be in pain or struggle? Why have poor quality sleep? Finding a balance between doing and being is the key to reaching your true potential with the career, lifestyle, and health you want.

To do this, you will first learn in this book what is occurring in your body, as you perceive one stressor after another. In addition, you will learn how you can live in the present more to empower your every thought, action, or word. Lastly, what steps you can take with a proven methodology that can bring you into harmonious balance, free of stress, worry, anxiety, chronic illness, insomnia, etc.

As a graduate student working toward a Ph.D. at Yale University, I remember seeing the difference between stress experienced as uncontrollable versus a stress that you can control. Yes, control is a central issue, as we will see again later, when it comes to overcoming stress. No, not control in an obsessive way, but control in the sense that you can change your relationship toward stressful situations and people.

All too often we blame the exterior (i.e., our spouse, boss, or a deadline) for our struggles or anxieties, but none of that is responsible, for the control lies within our own self. Once you let go of this outer control and devote more time to the anchor within, you will find that less of the noise and bustle outside will perturb your inner peace and joy, and you can remain tranquil, free, and highly productive.

I wrote this book because I do not want to see you struggle anymore. I want you to find the happiness and beauty within so that you may share it with your loved ones. I want to teach you how to live with laughter in your heart at all times, like an ageless child filled with bountiful excitement, love, and energy.

Yes, life is meant to be playful, even during difficult moments. You can master this art of playful living through your own self-efforts, though I can be by your side until you can do this on your own. I want you to learn how to tap into your own inner strength and your vast resources to better cope, manage, and conquer anything that may seem insurmountable at the start.

You have the blueprint already inside of you to become the architect of your own life and make significant growth and change in any arena of your life. All you may be missing are the lessons and principles that I am going to teach you in this book and possibly beyond the book as well. You already have all your dreams and goals inside of you. Let us work to bring these out now for you to live the way you want and deserve, free of stress, worry, or doubt, and full of passion, joy, and freedom. I know you can become the master of your dreams and your own reality.

Every moment can be a learning opportunity, and you deserve to take advantage of them. Know that you are exactly where you need to be. You should be proud of who you are and what you have accomplished thus far. However, you should never settle for less. Your loved ones deserve the best version of you, and I hope to humbly serve you to help you reach your highest potential.

This book is my first offering to you. I know that you can change your current circumstances and make them exactly what you choose to them to be. You can do this not by changing others or the outside first, but by starting with yourself, working from within and letting the new light that emerges color your exterior.

You deserve to take the time to heal, nurture, and strengthen yourself at the core. Yes, you may be busy, and feelings of guilt may creep up, but remember that you are not just doing this for yourself, you are also doing this for your partner and other loved ones.

Start by owning every moment that has led to this point, whether happy or sad, healthy or sick, whether you have lied or told the truth, or whether you have offended or hurt many or been a source of peace and love. It is not a coincidence that you are reading this book. There is a deeply meaningful relationship with the events that have brought you to this point and the words you now read.

I truly feel that, in a Jungian synchronicity kind of way, I was meant to join you on this journey at this very moment. If you approach this moment receptive to the grace that is being offered, then you can receive the healing currents contained within my own heart. Open your heart to these words and let them carry you until you may stand on your own two feet.

Loving kindness is the greatest healing tonic, and it is being offered to heal and nurture you. I know that you will find greater tranquility and freedom with time, patience, and perseverance. Do not, under any circumstances, give up, for you deserve to find your True Self in the here and now.

Together, I know we can get to the crux of the matter, to the heart of the problem. Soon you will realize that all I am doing at this moment is facilitating the release of the wisdom and love that already lies within you. You are consciousness, truth, beauty, and bliss. You do not need anything or anyone to have peace and love in your life. You do not need to be filled with love by another but can instead become a fountain of crystal-clear water waiting to burst forth to sustain others instead of waiting to be sustained. What gift then could you bestow on your loved ones in that scenario?

That is all you need, but the problem is how to get there. In this book, I begin to share some of the insights of more than two decades of scientific and yogic research to discover what lies behind the dreadful stress we so dislike. I will share how to overcome it and how to master the art of living a healthy and joyful life full of energy, vigor, and calmness that is not dependent on anything or anyone, and which you can then use to enhance all your relationships and endeavors in your life. You do not need to continue searching the exterior for more conditions that you think are crucial toward increasing your sense of happiness, such as money, a bigger house, fame, a stronger business, etc. You have everything you need right here and now.

Accept yourself as you are right here, at this moment, pain or no pain, fear or no fear, whether feeling strong or weak, confident or diffident. Treat yourself as a star actress playing your role and embrace it rather than shunning it. Say to yourself more often: "I can do this, I deserve better. I will do this for myself and then share it with my spouse and loved ones." Or "I am beautiful, strong, and brave." To neutralize negative ideology, as we will see in Chapter 11, we must counteract our pessimistic or unhealthy views with positive and enlightened words or affirmations.

In addition, after reading this book or working directly with me, you may find yourself thinking more often: "Here comes another stressful situation. Now is the time to tune into my breath and maintain awareness of the moment-to-moment changes occurring within and without me." And in this way, you can actively navigate through any situation that, in the past, would have swept you away.

Do not let anything or anyone take you away anymore. The world deserves to see your beauty, your love, and your greatness. These traits are built into the very fabric of your being but are veiled by different barriers and obstacles. Today is the day that you will take these barriers and obstacles down piece by piece, moment-to-moment, to begin to let the Real You shine through more and more.

You deserve that and more. That is my gift to you. I hope you can join me, and I promise that I will do my best to unwrap that gift with you to share with all your loved ones.

Like the Buddha, weep less and laugh more. Laughter is one of the greatest of all habits and is a gift you can share with anyone. It gives the right meaning to life and gives it the right color. Laughter can heal your body, lighten your burdens, and elevate your mood. It can sweep away the stresses of life in an instant, but only if you do it more often.

Let us try something before continuing further. Assume your favorite and most comfortable seated position. Take a moment before we continue to close your eyes for a few minutes and slow down your breathing. Make your breaths deep and long. As you sense your mind calming down as much as possible, visualize yourself as a child. See yourself in that child body moving through an open field. Notice yourself before the conditioned behaviors, habits, struggles, scars, sleepless nights, and traumas, whatever may have brought you to this point.

What attributes did you have that are now seemingly gone? Did you possess greater flexibility, peace of mind, gentleness, ability to sleep soundly and deeply, contentment, simplicity, curiosity, or capacity for playfulness and laughter? Have you lost or forsaken some of these attributes? Do you wish to rediscover and express them fully like before? Well, this book can help with that.

Using mainly yogic and Ayurvedic techniques, I will show you how you can rediscover the inner child to experience some of the joys and wonders of life again and recover the energy and health you once possessed before injuries, stress, injurious habits, etcetera stripped you of that.

Just as a yoga *asana* practice can bring your body to a more youthful state of flexibility and suppleness, other practices can help you to reclaim what is yours by birthright. You can radiate all those qualities I just mentioned and more. You can rediscover the playfulness, freedom, peace, and joy you once had, become free of stress and worry, and again find contentment and excitement in even the simplest of details, which will enhance your happiness, improve all your relationships, and even increase your productivity and success at work. Just as a child often brings the best out in others, so can you do the same.

May you rediscover the Real You, the Eternal Witness, who has been there all along, waiting to shine through all the numerous veils and obstacles you have put forth. May you break free from pain, disease, sleepless nights, stress, anxiety, fears, etc. This book is here to help make your life what you wish it to be and settle for nothing less. Both you and your loved ones deserve this.

You can make your life exactly what you wish it to be, just as an artist can fill a canvas with his or her own inner brilliance and creativity. Let us get the obstacles out of the way to allow your full expression to shine through, even in the midst of your own limitations or disabilities. I want to help you to discover the Master Artist that you already are so that you can begin to paint the canvas of your life with the colors of truth, love, health, happiness, beauty, radiance, and creativity!

Let us begin this journey. *Hari Om Tat Sat!*

Chapter 1:

Where did I go?

"Remember to look up at the stars and not down at your feet. Try to make sense of what you see and wonder about what makes the universe exist. Be curious. And however difficult life may seem, there is always something you can do, and succeed at. It matters that you don't just give up."

— Stephen Hawking

The bustle of the day is a whirlwind that sweeps you away through time. From the past, your mind flits briefly to the present, and then back to the past as you ruminate through one dead memory after another that only exists in your memory banks. With regret or longing, you enliven these dead memories in your mind's eye and may even feel guilty or sad about something you did or said, or something that was done or said to you. You may think about the so-called better days, when everything seems to have been happier. You confuse true happiness with a version that contains significant obstacles or conditions.

On more than one occasion, you may find yourself worrying about the future. What deadlines are looming at work? What bills do you have to pay this afternoon? Where do the children have to go after school on Tuesday? What will you make for dinner? This apparently endless to-do list may even fill you with dread or worry, fueling the fires of depression or anxiety.

You may think you are in the present moment as you do a task on the computer or a smartphone, cook, watch television, or drive hastily to work. However, you are just replacing one mind-occupying habit with another, expending enormous amounts of energy on these types of habits. This constant noise distracts you from the greatest gift you already possess, your True Self. This never-ending cycle begins soon after you wake up and sometimes even keeps you up at night, reducing your productivity and connectedness to others during the daytime, and even causing insomnia at bedtime.

Notice your mental state upon awakening, the calmness you may feel, the lessened thought waves, the worries that have not begun or the to-do list that has not yet come to the forefront of your mind. Become aware of how the noise inside builds as you go about your day. Try to stop yourself in your mental tracks and observe the processes that often consume the majority of your day and energy.

You replace one thought with another, rarely, if ever, controlling the inner chatter that invades your present and prevents you from being fully aware and alive in the moment. You do this all the time as you go about your duties. You may even talk or text on the phone in an effort to keep your mind busy and distracted. Rarely do you find time away from this process of doing, working, moving, and thinking.

This process is very energy-intensive and is not conducive to a state of inner peace and joyfulness. The habit of non-being that afflicts us all prevents you from relaxing in the present, where you could find true happiness and serenity. This constant activity does not allow your mind to dwell on a single point and empty itself. Thus, it prevents you from witnessing deeper aspects of yourself that can only be experienced in quiescence. You cannot easily enjoy the present moment or reduce thought vibrations that generate noise and agitate your mind vigorously unless you gain control over this process.

Your spouse, family members, or friends may have become accustomed to this version of you. You have lost sight of who you were before so many responsibilities, problems, and duties took over the bulk of your time and energy. You may struggle with anger at times, take out your frustration on those who love you, or build up tension in your body, causing pain or discomfort. Where have you gone? Indeed, you are often your own worst enemy.

With your busy and sometimes chaotic schedule, you rarely set aside the time to reclaim your True Self slowly, patiently, and lovingly by cultivating healthier habits, an optimistic view, increased adaptability, higher ethical standards that improve your relationship with yourself and others, and better awareness of not only your body, but also your mind. These and other factors can be integrated into your daily life with practice and perseverance so that you can become freer of stress, doubt, fear, and worry. You can also become free of mindlessness and full of mindfulness.

This and more can be yours, but what will you do about it? Will this just be one of the many self-help books you have read, or half-read? Will you seek out personal help from me or someone else, only to give up halfway and stay where you are?

Break the cycle and join me in this venture. There is a great voyage ahead, but it is only for those who are willing to let go and fly free. Your wings may have become clipped, but I know they can be healed, and that you can again learn how to soar high and far to reach the destiny you are meant to enjoy.

Something that I hope can become clear at some point during this journey together is that if you work on being mindful, stress will become a rarity. Focusing all your energies on a singular moment will set you free from worry about the future, doubt about yourself due to lack of focus and faith, and regret and longing for the past. The only thing you have is the eternal now. If all your energy is concentrated there, in that moment, everything becomes more vibrant, powerful, and rich, and you become truly free and boundless.

As your journey unfolds with the practices outlined ahead, notice how you cannot be stressed in the present. If you do not allow excessive energies condensed in the past, in the form of pervasive and dark memories, or bring from the future energy as worry or fantasy, you prevent your consciousness from being invaded and overwhelmed.

There is certainly an element of energy work and channeling that is involved in this process. I can teach you how to unlock this reserve of power asleep in most and learn how to use it to your advantage to avoid being run over by the energies all around you, especially those that we consider a threat to our well-being and peace of mind.

All too often you may find yourself adding conditions to your happiness, which will only prevent you from enjoying your life in the here and now. Why wait to be happy and at peace? Why wait until someone else changes, or you get the job you want, or your children are out of the house, or you can move into the house of your dreams, or your partner changes and becomes who you dream of, or you get the raise you want? None of these or any other events or acquisitions will ever bring true and lasting happiness.

The intention of this book is to be an invaluable resource that triggers an awakening into the present. Where you can break free from the culture of fast-paced living that our society nurtures. Where you can find the way to take better care of your body by reducing the many poisons or toxins that we often load up our body with, like stress, unhealthy dead food and habits, poor sleeping and breathing, lack of mindfulness, overworking ourselves without a proper counterbalance like relaxation, etc.

All I want is for you to train or teach yourself to stand on your own two feet and break this vicious cycle. To learn how to profit rather than deficit from your life, how to settle into being rather than just doing, how to breathe in a way that energizes you and brings peace and harmony, how to heal yourself through a multidimensional approach, how to love yourself, your life, your relationships, and your job unconditionally, etc.

Think about what will happen if you do not do anything right now, or if you do not get help. What will you be missing? Why not take the plunge and let go of fear, worry, or doubt? Is it really a coincidence that you are reading these words? There are no coincidences in life. Either you are in sync with the flow of life and using the resources given to your advantage, or you are missing out on one opportunity after another to discover your own innate greatness, your natural state of beauty, love, and bliss.

Do you really want this? Then read on and remain open, faithful, and sincere. Listen with your heart and have confidence that only truthful words and advice is soon to follow. A life of love and service is poured into this book. May you reap the benefits it is designed to unfold. I see in you a perfectly adorned gift waiting to be opened, revealing the greatest gift this world has ever seen, the Real You.

Know you are loved and not alone, even if sometimes it seems like you are. Together, I know we can do this. You can uncover the contents of that most prized gift. Do your partner, family, children, or friends not deserve to see that? Do you not deserve that as well?

Breaking It Down

To begin this journey, in Chapter 3, I will describe the ins and outs of stress, summarizing what I have learned after nearly two decades of research, practice, and reflection. What are some of its physiological effects or causes? How does this affect our nervous and endocrine systems? What is the relationship between stress and a number of chronic ailments? The goal in this chapter will not be to burden you with what is wrong about stress and your health, but to give you better insight and perspective that will give you the power to do something before it is too late. It is imperative that you are well-informed and can make wise, conscientious decisions.

With that information, in Chapter 4 we will begin to learn how to care for your body to increase energy, vitality, and health. In Appendix B, I will share some additional nutritional secrets to avoid health-related or body-associated stress and inflammation. If we do not do anything, the body will continue to be an obstacle to rediscovering the calmness, longevity, and peace you can share with your loved ones.

Another topic that is important and will be emphasized throughout the book, especially in Chapter 5, is balance. I will not take lightly how to achieve this balance when faced with daily stressors. Remaining balanced, even when faced with extreme adversity, is under your control.

We will continue to build toward a comprehensive and holistic approach in Chapter 6 by teaching you how to be your own healer by helping you reconnect with your body, mind, and spirit, beginning with the body. By reconnecting with your body, you can identify where stress is stored as excess energy, how you are holding on to it, and how to let go. Therapeutic yoga techniques, yoga *nidra* (conscious sleep or relaxation), and body scanning are some of the methods that will be shared, along with Ayurvedic self-massage and how to properly practice *asana* (yoga postures) for stress relief and as a natural conduit to meditation.

Not only is it important for you to learn the different practices to do at home, but it is equally as important for you to know how to take these practices outside and into the real world. What use is it if you spend eight to ten hours outside of your house and cannot be shown how to integrate your practice at work, for example? I want you to be mindful and present at all times, if possible. In this way, you maintain a healing and nurturing mental attitude throughout the day. The stress of work can be one of the most crippling for some. Thus, our relationship with work becomes a key factor when managing stress, as we will see in Chapter 7. If our livelihood is not our passion, then we must make time for our passions outside of work on a regular basis.

I also want you to discover how to tap into your natural state of inner peace and how to carry that throughout the day and into the night. As we will see in Chapter 8, stress often leads to insomnia or poorer quality of sleep due to an inability to maintain a particular state of restorative rest. I will share simple techniques and approaches that can improve your ability to sleep and the quality of that sleep.

In Chapter 9, we will see how time can be one of our biggest enemies, as our culture is always in a rush to do more and more in less time. You can discover how to slow down time, concentrate more, and do more in less time. In addition, I want you to learn how to take time for yourself in a guilt-free way, since you are not doing this just for you but also for those around you, including your partner or loved ones.

As we progress, we will touch upon a number of different topics mostly from a yogic point of view. One of these is *santosha,* or contentment. In Chapter 10, we will see how much of our stress originates from seeking outwardly for praise or reward and feeling unsatisfied with our current role or life circumstances. Know that you matter and are beautiful just the way you are. You are already happy and free but need only to realize it in the here and now. Believe in yourself more and have faith that you are exactly where you should be. You should do your duties with care and love, but not forget that you can always work to improve your current circumstances, not by viewing them negatively or getting frustrated, but by getting organized and focused and putting your time, energy, money, and effort into getting where you want.

Then we get to Chapter 11, which may very well be one of the most important chapters, as we will safeguard you against yourself. There are hidden dimensions of your consciousness that can pose problems and become obstacles. Learning how to combat these unseen forces will be key. Negative ideology is at the top of the list, as it often leads us to do the opposite of what is in our best interest. It is what saps us of much-needed energy to do what will bring us into balance. To this end, positive and powerful affirmations, mantras, and mindfulness meditation can help to free you from these forces and help you to reclaim your free will. Changing your perspective on the source of your problems and your stress will be discussed, as it does not lie at all outside of you, but within yourself.

Lastly, in Chapter 12, I want to share how to take it to the next level and put it all together consistently. You know you want to make changes, and it starts now. If long-term success is your main goal, as it should be, then I am here to help establish a program based on your needs, your past, and your distinct plan of development and growth. I want you to discover why you are here, where you are going, and what are you meant to do in this lifetime. That discovery will bring a great sense of meaning and joy to your life and that of others around you as well. Are you ready to begin? If so, let's move on and learn why I wrote this book, and about stress and how to make it an ally.

Chapter 2:

Why I Wrote This Book

"Happiness cannot come from without. It must come from within.
It is not what we see and touch or that which others do for us
which makes us happy; it is that which we think and feel and do,
first for the other fellow and then for ourselves."

— Helen Keller

My Wife as the Channel

I wrote this book in honor of my loving wife, Norma, to whom I have dedicated this book, and who is at the heart of many of the successes in my life. We have been married for more than eleven years. Her sacrifices have, in many ways, made this book possible. For nearly two decades, I had wanted to share the ideas contained herein, but it was not until now that everything fell into place and, through her undying support, this book became possible.

For far too long, I have seen Norma be a hero to this household but rarely realize it, as she often waited for acknowledgments and affirmations from others that she was what we all knew: amazing, kind, giving, talented, loving, and strong. During this time, I have seen her struggle on and off with chronic stress, anxiety, panic attacks, and depression.

Norma would fight through many a difficult moment like a fierce warrior, but often not recover well, to the point where it has weakened her will and her health over the years. For far too long, I have seen her, like many others, look without for happiness rather than within.

I know I was not always there the way she needed, as I myself had my own struggles of maturation and dealing with responsibilities. In addition, I was viewing her struggles from my point of view and not hers. I realized that, when trying to connect with and help someone, you have to meet others where they are first and not treat them as if they already knew what you were trying to share.

Society and maybe even your own family have a way of focusing on what is wrong with you, what we project or express. However, that is not the real you. I want you to know that I see so much beauty, love, and bliss already there, present and available. Why not take steps to let that come out more and touch those around you, especially your loved ones, like the warm hand of a mother caressing her baby? Let them witness your inner light shining through.

I believe in you, and together we can rediscover the innate calmness, balance, and freedom you once enjoyed as a child when you were full of vibrancy, curiosity, joy, and wonder. Life has a way of putting us down, of presenting us with many an obstacle that we do not often handle well.

In the process, we can lose ourselves as we continue onward on the path set before us. However, that is not the only avenue we can take. We can, in the here and now, reshape and restructure our entire life starting with the very fabric of our own being by rediscovering our True Self deep within, hiding like a scared, lost child. Together, we can nurture that inner child with a profound love and a deep understanding that is based on solid research and applied evidence.

Thus, I have written this book as a service to anyone who wants to integrate into their lives some of the secrets shared within these pages. It is my hope as well that Norma will integrate what is shared in this book by putting into practice the lessons and techniques described. In a way, Norma is essential to help breathe life into a journey of service and love.

I do not want to see Norma, or anyone else, struggle through life being anything other than the best version of themselves. I want her to find the happiness and beauty that lies within us all and to be able to share it with anyone. I want her to find freedom from stress and conflict by experiencing union through love so that any relationship can flourish. I know without a shadow of a doubt that if she does, others will find it too. Norma, in a way my ideal reader, will help to bridge the gap between my love for service and spiritual illumination and those craving its most precious gifts.

Path to Service

Even as a child and adolescent, I experienced, through the eyes of others, the ravages of stress-induced problems. I grew up in a household where my mother struggled with the stresses of everyday life (i.e., working, raising kids, managing a household, cooking for us, taking care of my father, etc.). At an early age, I saw through her how a lack of control would tip her over the edge. She struggled with emotions, especially anger and anxiety, and it got worse for a time after she and my dad got divorced. Those emotions got transferred to us as kids, and as an adult, I could see how all that energy from the past would come out in the present. I could feel her anger or her anxiety as I encountered my own difficulties as a parent and husband.

It is not surprising to me then, that, at a young age, I was attracted to the topic of mental health issues. I always had a deep fascination with the brain and deeper aspects of the Self. I loved to watch human behavior and dynamics, what made people respond the way they did or make the decisions that, for better or worse, would drive their destiny in one direction or another.

Those experiences and many others attracted me to Yale University and the Department of Neurobiology and, even earlier, lead me to a nonprofit

Spiritist center in Puerto Rico, Instituto de Cultura Espirita Renacimiento, where I served to heal, with the help of others, many people suffering from a variety of physical, mental, and spiritual conditions. It was at that Institute that I began to see the potential inherent in humans, the power of latent psychic abilities, and the vast dimensions of consciousness untapped or unrealized by most.

Those untapped or unrealized dimensions are at the heart of who we are and how we experience the present. I discovered early on that, to achieve enlightenment and peace, one had to conquer the dark and dense formations embedded in our psyche. I knew that, to help enhance my understanding and effectively help others, I needed to start my career studying the nervous system, which allows us to express ourselves on the physical plane of existence.

Therefore, after graduating from the University of Puerto Rico, I moved to New Haven, CT, to begin a doctorate program in Neurobiology at Yale University. There, I hoped to begin putting the pieces together by learning about the nervous system and how we are connected, as infinite spirits, to the body.

I had a deep interest in mental health and for some time, thought about going to medical school to help improve the field of psychiatry, which I felt was sorely in need of a more holistic approach to multidimensional beings like humans. However, I decided that I could make more of an impact by using my expertise and experience to promote change with my work, passion, and writings outside of the field of psychiatry.

During graduate school and even after obtaining a Ph.D., I immersed myself for years in the study of the effects of stress on the nervous and endocrine systems and how this would influence our health. I became deeply interested in the subject of how we could influence our gene expression with our habits, conduct, experiences, etc., and even how mental control originating from within could abolish most, if not all, of the effects of stress, even those at a genetic or cellular level. In the process, a person could become free of disease, anxiety, worry, or fear.

I also rediscovered yoga and Ayurveda in my early twenties, which provided me with a clearer vision of how to reign in our thought waves and our energies to increase our vitality, power, and strength of will. I found in yoga an experiential methodology, similar to the scientific process, that could help bring anyone back to their native state of happiness, freedom, and bliss, which they once enjoyed at an early age. Yoga and many valuable suggestions and techniques described in this book, when practiced as I describe them, could help bring a person back to a more youthful and joyous time as an ageless child free from the constraints of time and space, death and disease.

I pursued the path of Self-Realization through advanced yogic practices for many years to rediscover this state and be able to convey it to the serious student. Despite this, I soon realized that I could not continue further without helping others realize it themselves as well. Going within was not that valuable without the complementary component of loving service unto others.

Moreover, I had been a successful westerner, who had studied at an Ivy League school, written numerous scientific publications, started various businesses, raised a family, lost a parent at an early age, and been through many a stressful moment. Yet, I had discovered during those two decades or so these vast realms of consciousness untapped by most and described by many a sage or master of yore.

I knew that my destiny led to healing others and then serving as a guide to awaken and help them Self-Realize as well, to attain true freedom and immortality, endless peace, and indescribable bliss. I had no doubt that anyone could achieve that state if offered the right path, starting first with a holistic healing approach that can unlock powerful transpersonal growth and evolution.

Therefore, I began a process of deep introspection and analysis, of searching for the very best in the healing arts and enlightenment, never settling for anything less than the truth, the best methodology, process, habit, tool, or technique. I was determined to integrate and put into practice anything that I knew would later help others improve their own condition, health, stability, and even spiritual advancement.

Some may have thought that I was doing this for myself, but in fact, all along, I had humanity and its suffering in the forefront of my mind. All I could ever hope for and dream of would be to become the purest expression of truth, consciousness, and bliss (*satchitananda*) and offer it to anyone receptive enough to receive it.

I believed back then, and thereafter confirmed, that there was a long-term solution to chronic physical and mental care and to stress-related conditions. You can, through natural and self-driven means, gain relief from life's many ailments, no matter the current condition you find yourself in.

Humanity is moving steadily into an era of holistic, natural, and spiritual pathways to health, longevity, and wellness, with results that stay with you for longer periods and free you from dependency on medications or at the very least reduce their intake. We can become stress-, worry-, disease-, and pain-free by taking the necessary steps with the right tools and help.

It was with these sincere intentions and love that this book came to be. After quite a voyage, the book has finally arrived in the present, and I hope that it can touch your life and help you find greater health, happiness, freedom, and peace.

Chapter 3:

What is Stress?

"Fight or flight? If I had wings, there'd be no choice.
But since I don't have wings, I have to rely on my cape,
and a long running start."

— Jarod Kintz

As a Ph.D. with a strong background in the neurosciences and mental health, I feel I need to explain what stress is and how it can be affecting you before we jump into solutions. You need to understand what you are dealing with to effectively and consciously change what contributes to your stress-related problems.

Stress is the silent killer of our generation, and we cannot assume that we are okay just because a disease has not struck, we think we are doing well at work, we feel we are making enough money, or we are managing with a version of ourselves that is less than ideal, even if it is accepted by those close to us. Therefore, bear with me as we navigate through this chapter. I promise that the rest of the book goes into how to deal with stress and its varied effects (from overcoming illness, anxiety, or pain or improving sleep). If any question may arise related to the concepts in this chapter, please feel free to reach out to me as a friend on social media, as I am here to serve in any way you may need.

Danger: Real or Illusion?

As you navigate through the world, your body is sensing its environment and asking itself in a way, "Am I in danger? Is my survival at risk?" If the answer is no, then everything is business as usual and you remain calm and focused on whatever you were doing. However, if the answer is yes, then the body will quickly respond to either a real physical threat (i.e., a wild animal ready to pounce or a car accident) or, what is more common for us, a psychological or psychosocial stimulation that arises from your own mental or emotional responses to what otherwise should be neutral and uneventful.

You do not live in danger all the time. In fact, humans rarely encounter dangerous situations, yet many of us turn on the stress pathway for purely psychological or psychosocial reasons. Today, you do not turn the street corner and encounter a wild animal pouncing to bite you. Because of this, you should not have your stress pathways activated as often as you do. You live like a gazelle in the savannah, when in fact you are a human living in a protected and safe environment.

Despite living in this way, you stress out due to other stimuli of a purely psychological nature, often with no direct physical stressor. These psychological stressors are highly dependent on how you perceive and process them. Examples of these types of stressors include deadlines at work, an upcoming test, a failing marriage, a sick relative who you need to care for, etc. Often these events or people in your life put a lot of pressure on you. You feel on a day-to-day basis that you have responsibilities that you are obligated to fulfill and that you need to produce more than your natural capacity allows for.

Therefore, the way you go about your life favors the activation of stress pathways in your body with its related global, physiological response mediated by nervous and endocrine structures, with specific neurochemicals and hormones, respectively. What we humans show is an anticipatory stress-response. If there is no actual physical stressor yet you routinely anticipate it, then you enter the realm of mental health problems that have become so pervasive in our modern society, such as anxiety, neurosis, paranoia, or hostility. Moreover, our inability to relax and unwind in healthy ways keeps our body saturated with toxic levels of stress hormones and neurochemicals. You may not know this, but even animals take time to rest and relax, often much more than we do!

Whether you are in your household cleaning, paying the bills, taking care of your children, working at a job you dislike, running a large corporation, being a workaholic, or even being unable to pay your mortgage, these all increase your stress levels due to chronic psychological stress. Your to-do list has no end, and, if you are not organized, this list can overwhelm you at times.

You are likely stuck in a near perpetual state of doing, having lost sight of simply being and enjoying yourself and your loved ones. You may find it difficult, if not impossible, to relax. Even when you think you are relaxing, you are still doing! This, of course, produces a significant and oftentimes crippling stress response that will inevitably catch up with you at some point. Since your stress response is not designed for these repeated psychological triggers without adequate relaxation, your disease risk increases, as we will see.

We live in a time where it has become increasingly rare to find people getting sick or dying of infectious diseases, poor hygiene, or malnutrition. Instead, thanks to the many advances of modern medicine, we live well and long enough to often encounter diseases of a more chronic nature, such as diabetes, cancer, heart disease, and neurodegeneration, all of which have connections to stress.

Our westernized lifestyle can be caused or worsened by stress. In fact, close to eighty percent of all doctor visits in the United States are related to stress and account for the third highest health-related expenditures. Therefore, it is of the utmost importance that you get to know stress and over-come its slow and silent inner workings, which can reduce the quality of your life. If you leave it to your doctor to educate you and help you, you will be left with the short end of the stick, as only three percent of doctors talk to patients about stress reduction practices or techniques.

Under normal circumstances, stress is an ally that helps an organism find the energy to reestablish homeostasis or balance, but, as you will see, chronic and unpredictable stress moves your body away from homeostasis and into the realm of pathological responses. Therefore, stress provides you with a great example of the mind-body connection, as your thoughts arising in another dimension can, through the nervous and endocrine systems, impact your body and health.

The physiological response to stress seems to originate in the limbic system of the brain, which regulates primitive behaviors or instincts. The limbic system, and in particular a structure called the hypothalamus, is the bridge, or axis, connecting higher cortical function with a physiological response (i.e., the fight-or-flight response seen during acute stress). Let us examine how this works, so that you can be well informed as to the dynamics of stress effects in your body both short- and long-term.

Getting to Know Stress

Stress is the response of the body to the events of life that you perceive as dangerous, harmful, or unable to be controlled. You could also define stress as a reaction to imminent and real danger, like when you are driving your car and almost get into an accident. Somebody cuts in front of your vehicle and this leads to the activation of an instinctual, physiological response you call stress, and scientists call the "fight-or-flight" response.

This response can manifest not only during extreme survival conditions, but also during events that you either mentally or emotionally react to with fear or lack of control, as if the situation was in fact an imminent danger or threatening. Whenever you experience an event in your life as going beyond your limits or capacity for control, the result is a feeling of adversity, hopelessness, or danger, even if unconsciously, that can trigger a response similar to the "fight-or-flight" response and involve the same neuroendocrine mechanism (i.e., adrenaline – or epinephrine – release).

Stress augments the functioning of specific systems of your body for a short- or long-term period. For example, stress mobilizes energy reserves for your neuromusculature, increases your heart rate for better transport of oxygen, and decreases blood flow to the digestive system. All these changes would be of value during a stressful, life-threatening event. The power of the "fight or flight" response is evident in the following examples.

In 2012, a twenty-two-year-old woman was able to lift a BMW car when the vehicle fell from a jack onto her father.[1] A few years later, a man was able to lift a Chevy Camaro to free a trapped cyclist in Arizona.[2] Lastly, a woman was able to wrestle a polar bear away from her son who was playing hockey with his friends in Quebec when attacked.[3]

As these examples illustrate, stress can help us to achieve superhuman feats, mainly through the activation of the sympathetic nervous system (SNS) by releasing adrenaline. The person in that moment is channeling the energy toward the neuromusculature to achieve powerful feats of power. Therefore, stress can be a source of immense power, but if it is not channeled correctly or if it is exposed to chronic, high levels of these chemicals, stress can lead to negative health consequences for both body and mind, as we will see.

Sympathetic vs. Parasympathetic Nervous System

The lack of balance in your life due mainly to stress involves two neurophysiological responses related to the SNS and the parasympathetic nervous system (PNS). These are part of the autonomic, or involuntary, nervous system, as opposed to your somatic, or voluntary, nervous system. The SNS mainly governs arousal and activity, while PNS activation enhances relaxation and rejuvenation. A balance between the activities of these two systems is crucial to your health and well-being.

Typically, the "fight-or-flight" response involves the activation of the SNS and a suppression of PNS activation. The stress response is not something negative, since it does provide the person with a number of benefits when activated acutely and for a specific purpose. For example, if I am exercising and my SNS does not increase my heart rate,[4] expand the air passages for more oxygenation,[5] and alter blood pressure to divert energy away from digestive system and toward the muscles,[6,7] I would be in trouble. This can happen very quickly mediated by adrenaline, also called epinephrine.

Without the SNS, you would have a difficult time getting out of bed, finding the energy to do things. In yoga, this system is related to right nostril breathing and to the spiritual quality called *rajas* (activation, agitation, energy, and movement). When you demonstrate sympathetic dominance, you breathe mostly through your right nostril and you show a tendency toward *rajas*. Of course, there is nothing wrong with this, as you need *rajas* to do things, to be active and energetic, and move with vigor and power. If you want to establish a morning practice, but energy is lacking, then you can do specific breathing techniques to energize yourself and counteract lethargy and inertia, known as the spiritual quality of *tamas*.

The PNS, on the other hand, mediates the opposite effect, inducing relaxation, a slower heart rate, stimulation of digestion and glandular activity, and helping to conserve energy. This system would be important at night when you need to relax, and you do not want to be overstimulated by too much energy or *rajas* circulating through your body. This system is related in yoga to the left nostril and to the spiritual quality of *tamas* (lethargy and inertia). Thus, when there is parasympathetic dominance, the left nostril passageway is more open, and you breathe more through it.

Interestingly, when you inhale and hold your breath, the SNS is stimulated, which is related to energy, morning practice, overcoming lethargy, etc. Conversely, when you exhale, your PNS is stimulated and it induces relaxation and sleepiness, allowing for rest and rejuvenation. However, with a dysfunctional PNS due to chronic stress, relaxation does not occur as effectively as before, and your heart rate remains elevated, for example. Your heart then works overtime.

Normally, it should increase its rate, as when you exercise, and then decrease when you stop and PNS kicks in. However, this acceleration and brake response becomes impaired over time.

Relaxation techniques described later in the book will emphasize balancing the SNS and PNS, and increasing PNS during times of stress, anxiety, worry, or panic. These techniques tend to augment the activity of the PNS, helping to reverse stress effects.[8] Chronic stress can lead to suboptimal levels of activity of the PNS and make it more difficult for you to relax, quiet your mind, and even sleep. Having too much PNS stimulation, however, is not ideal either because it will increase confusion, lethargy, drowsiness, and even induce depressive-like symptoms. Note how this is the opposite of SNS and *rajas*, which would increase arousal, energy, activity, and induce anxious-type symptoms.

Therefore, balance between the activation of these systems is crucial for mental and physical health. What you want is a balance between *rajas* and *tamas*, which leads to the perfect expression of both, and to the spiritual quality of *satvas* (harmony, serenity, peacefulness, etc.). This *sattvic* state is what you should seek to create and express more. Therefore, I devote various chapters to help teach you how to enhance its expression.

Prefrontal Cortex: Acute Response

In addition, within the nervous system, stress will turn off your frontal lobe, specifically the prefrontal cortex (PFC), which is a region of your brain that makes you human and inhibits instinctual and primitive regions of your brain.[9] Therefore, when the PFC is turned off, it switches your behavior to a more automatic and instinctual response.[10]

Let us again use the example of driving your car, when someone crosses in front of you, and you almost get in an accident. How does your body respond at that moment? Your heart starts to beat faster to mobilize the blood throughout the body and deliver energy more quickly. Energy stores are hydrolyzed, releasing glucose into the bloodstream in large amounts. Your heart rate increases to deliver energy and oxygen to your cells more quickly. You turn off your digestive tract (i.e., your mouth gets dry when stressed as secretions like saliva cease). You shut down growth and reproduction. Your immune system's function is enhanced but only acutely. There is suppression of pain (stress-induced analgesia just in case you are injured and need to ignore the pain). There is increased oxygenated blood and glucose to your brain, to enhance your senses and recall in the short-term, and so that you can very quickly or impulsively react to a dangerous or stressful situation. Blood is diverted from the core of your body and digestive system to your arms and legs, for example, to get out of the way of the car and to press the brake pad.

In addition to many of the physiological changes mediated by adrenaline, the areas of your brain that are active at that moment change, which is a crucial aspect of the stress response often ignored by laypeople. Your PFC, which is important for impulse control, measured and appropriate responses, and working memory, is turned off by the release in this region of large amounts of neuromodulators, like norepinephrine and dopamine.

Instead, other areas of the brain become active, like limbic areas of the hippocampus and amygdala, which are more automatic and instinctual areas of the brain and are what you need to be functioning at a high level in that moment. These areas will allow you to react quickly to imminent danger without the need to have to plan or reason through your actions or decisions. You can react quickly, impulsively, and instinctively in order to avoid danger and survive.

Despite these short-term benefits of stress, chronic activation of the stress response is detrimental to your health in ways you do not easily notice. For example, your body chronically ignores repair, planning for the future is affected as your prefrontal cortex atrophies, and wear and tear progresses without the much-needed periods of rest, healing, and regrowth, amongst many other changes detailed shortly.

When you enter a state of stress, levels of various neurochemicals, in particular neuromodulators that regulate brain function increase. This acute response to stress is what happens during the fight-or-flight response. In your life, this may be felt if your A/C breaks down, you have an emergency deadline at work, you just got in a fight with your partner, etc. In addition, there is also a more long-term component (see below) that affects the secretion of hormones called glucocorticoids, like cortisol, that are released by the adrenal gland. In this case, it may be due to dealing with sick family member, a divorce with children involved, or a failing business.

Long-term Response and Adaptation

The second component to stress and the one more relevant to our long-term health involves the hormone cortisol, a glucocorticoid. Cortisol will mobilize cells to start releasing energy into the bloodstream in the form of glucose to give your body what it needs when faced with a stressor. However, cortisol can also enter cells, like your brain cells or neurons, and bind to receptor proteins to act like a transcription factor, which changes your gene expression and the proteins your cells make.[11]

This of course will have clear advantages because, due to exposure to stress, cells can change and adapt to the tense or difficult situation the body is undergoing. Despite helping you adapt to these stressful situations, what happens if you are activating these pathways too often?

This is very similar to how drugs work. If you chronically use a drug, then you are changing your body over a long-term period, and your cells genetically change to adapt to the addiction. Drugs often augment the signaling of chemicals in your body, mostly in the nervous system. A signaling pathway, in a similar way to cortisol, will alter your gene expression and the proteins being produced and thus adapt you better to the addiction.[12] Chronic stress works in a similar way by increasing the release of neurochemicals and hormones at levels that cause adaptive or, worse yet, maladaptive changes in a way that is not healthy long-term, as we will see shortly.

In summary, so far, we have seen that stress has two components, one of which is the short-term component that acts very rapidly and powerfully and is mediated mainly by adrenaline, and another that is due to repeated bouts of stress without periods of rest and relaxation during our waking hours, which involves glucocorticoids like cortisol. Both of these forms of stress lead to physiological responses that can change your body in significant ways, whether quickly or worse, over the course of years.

The Biology of Being Frazzled[13]

So far, I have discussed the short-term effects of adrenaline. Let us now talk about noradrenaline and dopamine, mentioned briefly above. These are neuromodulators and, unlike neurotransmitters, do not activate neurons but modulate their activity, making them more or less responsive and thus able, for example, to impair the functioning of the prefrontal cortex during stressful periods.

The prefrontal cortex is a very important brain structure and is what makes us human in many respects. This region is very important for impulse control, emotional regulation, working memory (a form of short-term memory you use all the time), attention, etc. It is also a region that humans recently acquired in evolution and is still being perfected. Thus, it takes effort to use the prefrontal regions efficiently. This is why it is vulnerable to stress. In animals, not surprisingly, this lobe is much smaller in size and thus animals are much more impulsive and have a hard time regulating their primitive behaviors, being altruistic, and doing what is right yet difficult.

Working memory is what allows you, for example, to be able to hold on-line in the present the memory of what you just read, so that when you read the next sentence, you can put the two together into one cohesive thought or idea. This type of memory is what allows you to do work, to remember where you parked your car in the morning, etc. It is the ability of the prefrontal cortex, in many respects, that is at the heart of overcoming stress because it is crucial to being present, grounded, and attentive during your day-to-day activities and increasing concentration and mindfulness.

A strong prefrontal cortex will keep you focused on what matters, which is the eternal now of the present that is the only thing you truly have. If you want to be successful, yet your mind drifts into the past or future without control, then your prefrontal cortex activity is not going to be high and other more primitive areas of the brain will dominate your behavior and cognition. As you will see later on, it is in the realm outside of the present where often the problems lie and where stress can really take hold and run your life awry.

So why does the prefrontal cortex go off-line when exposed to stress? Acute stress causes neurons in the brainstem, those at the base of the brain above the spinal cord that produce the neuromodulators like dopamine and norepinephrine, to become more active. The activity of these neuromodulatory neurons leads to the release of higher levels than is optimal of norepinephrine and dopamine, which leads to prefrontal cortical dysfunction. These high levels of norepinephrine or dopamine effectively take the prefrontal cortex offline.

Alternatively, if you do not release enough of these neuromodulators, you can also take the prefrontal cortex offline. Thus, in what will be the hallmark of this book and especially of Chapter 5, you need balance.

Again, you see this accelerator and brake system. However, it is more than that. These neuromodulators demonstrate an inverted U response where both low levels of release as in fatigue, drowsiness, or depression (excessive *tamas*), or high levels as with uncontrollable stress (excessive *rajas*) lead to impairment of prefrontal cortical functioning. Only with balanced or moderated levels of release can the prefrontal cortex work optimally to enhance attention, working memory, impulse control, mindfulness, etc.[14]

In this way, you can remain more focused at work and at home. Additionally, you can begin to show a better, happier side of yourself, have less fits of anger or impatience, let go of the noise that disturbs your peace of mind and interrupts your sleep, and maintain your composure and calmness, even when faced with adversity. Finally, you can enhance your meditative or yogic practices further to prepare you better for the path toward Self-Realization.

Cortisol: Long-term Adaption and Disease

I have talked about the short-term effects of stress, which are immediate and powerful. However, the long-term effects of stress are likely the most pernicious to our overall health and well-being. Our exposure to so many daily different sources of intermittent and unpredictable stressors adds up over time to culminate in a state of chronic stress that involves slower changes within our cells through an alteration in gene expression, as mentioned previously.

The nervous system again plays a crucial role through two brain structures called the hypothalamus and pituitary gland, collectively called the hypothalamic-pituitary axis (HPA). When exposed to stress, whether physical or psychological, the hypothalamus releases corticotropic releasing hormone (CRH), which causes pituitary cells to release adrenocorticotropic releasing hormone (ACTH). ACTH travels through the bloodstream to the adrenal cortex of the adrenal gland, where it leads to the release of a key glucocorticoid involved in the stress response called cortisol.

Cortisol, as I have mentioned before, helps make the stress response beneficial under acute circumstances by mobilizing sugar (glucose) in the bloodstream, for example. However, cortisol can also have negative effects on the body. Long-term exposure to higher than normal levels of cortisol, as happens with chronic stress, can change the gene expression in many of our cells including in the brain.[15,16,17] This is the adaptive process to stress that can atrophy certain brain regions (i.e., hippocampus), impair long-term memory, increase our risk of certain diseases, and affect our mood or mental health.

If you are not under real danger that requires the activation of a survival, instinctual, physiological, and behavioral response, why would you want these genetic processes activated? You do not deserve to live with the alarm on all the time, like if the alarm in your house were on constantly even though there is no risk of a burglar breaking in. That noise over time would drive you crazy! It is like that for many of us: living with constant noise, filling it with more stress and more noise.

We are constantly doing, without learning the necessary balance of settling the mind and enjoying just being, empty from the thoughts, worries, and stressors of everyday life. It is okay to want to be powerful and successful in your business or career, yet you must leave time to empty yourself to promote healing, clarity, and great enjoyment of the present moment, and to be able to reach deeper, more profound states of consciousness that lead to true freedom and endless bliss.

In addition, living in a state of alarm or alert all the time is very unhealthy to your mind and body. This is very important to understand. Take a military lifestyle, especially during moments of war and even during basic training, where the alarm needs to be on often; you see many cases of psychiatric problems related to frontal lobe dysfunction.

Cortisol, like I mentioned above, can modify your gene expression and modify the structure of your neurons.[18] If you examine the brain (i.e., hippocampus or prefrontal cortex) of someone with high levels of cortisol, you will see clear structural abnormalities often associated with: (1) deficits in brain function, (2) neuropsychiatric problems, (3) poor working memory and long-term memory, (4) poor attention, (5) impulse and emotional control issues, (6) decreased neurogenesis or growth and development of new neural tissue, etc. You may think that you do not show most, if any, of these deficits or problems, however, you are likely operating at less than peak level in many, if not all, all of these.

Chronic Stress and Diabetes

Since stress through cortisol release mobilizes glucose in the bloodstream,[19] it also indirectly increases levels of insulin, the hormone that causes cells to take in glucose to lower sugar levels in the blood. Chronically diverting energy from storage sites inside cells and releasing it into the bloodstream, only to store it again, disrupts this key biochemical process over time and increases the risk of metabolic diseases such as diabetes.

Indeed, chronic stress complicates sugar regulation and can contribute to diabetes-like symptoms or exacerbate an already expressed diabetes type-2. It can push the body to greater insulin resistance and thus sugar levels can remain higher.

How can this happen? Well, hyperglycemia (high sugar in blood) triggers increased insulin release. As insulin is released in high amounts more often to control blood sugar levels, insulin can cause a down regulation of its receptor. With less insulin receptors to respond with, cells do not take up glucose as efficiently.[20,21] It is like the cell senses too much insulin stimulation and removes its receptor. This is how insulin-resistant type-2 diabetes could be exacerbated or complicated. With less receptors for insulin, cells just do not take up glucose as efficiently when released during stress, and sugar levels can remain higher for longer. Cortisol is involved in this process and is a complicating factor for diabetes.[22]

Chronic Stress and Cancer

Glucocorticoids, like cortisol, can act as immunosuppressors[23] and thus can make us more vulnerable to many common diseases, such as cold or flu. Potentially worse than these diseases, is the link of chronic stress to cancer, in animal studies in particular. High levels of stress and glucocorticoids in animals causes tumors already present to grow faster and increases the risk of relapse.

Although these studies are controversial due to the ambiguity of the results in human studies, it is at least likely that stress hormones increase the risk for getting cancer. Chronic stress alone, however, despite leading to immunosuppression, is not enough to cause cancer or even influence its progression because the immunosuppression is not large enough.

However, it does make sense that a weakened immune system will not be as successful at detecting abnormal cancer cells and killing them, allowing them to flourish long enough to become a bigger problem. It has become clear that stress and cortisol at the very least can lead to fatigue, depression, and dissipation of energy, which reduces the functioning of the body and accelerating the progression of diseases like cancer, as some studies suggest.[24]

Despite all this, more research is needed, and we are not at a point where anyone should sell a stress reduction program as a remedy for cancer. It does not hurt as an adjunct treatment, but it should not be the only step taken to fight cancer. Just like with any suggestion given in this book, working with your doctor(s) is always of importance.

Chronic Stress and Alzheimer's Disease

Stress can interact with our genes, as I have mentioned previously, and activate pathways that should not be on in adulthood. When I was at Yale, I saw the parallels between stress pathways inside the cells and neurodegenerative conditions like Alzheimer's disease. Although it is still too early to tell, some early indications are that chronic stress in middle age could cause dementia in later life.[25] Animal studies for sure demonstrate a link between stress hormones and memory impairment that is a hallmark of Alzheimer's disease.[26]

Chronic Stress and Psychiatric Illness

Some final examples of the silent workings of stress and cortisol include the following. Firstly, the presence of a significant stressor or treatment with glucocorticoids, like cortisol, for an extended period correlates with risk for early-stage depression. Glucocorticoids also act on the amygdala and increase fear and anxiety. Chronic intermittent periods of stress over-stimulate the SNS, leading to a number of physical and mental ailments, such as irritable bowel syndrome or anxiety disorders. Lastly, chronic stress, in contrast to what moderate stress does, depletes us of dopamine, the neuromodulator that increases our pleasure and motivation, which can lead to addiction relapse or taking a drug more to boost dopamine levels.

Final Thoughts

It has become clear that chronic stress can increase the risk of a number of physical and mental conditions due to decreased disease resistance.

Chronic diseases associated with stress, and seen more often nowadays, are the slow and silent killers of our generation, often causing or exacerbating diseases that are present at subtle or mental levels way before they manifest physically. Even when they are manifesting physically, they may not be perceived and can carry over time and worsen with continued exposure to stress, poor diet, and other factors.

These stress-related diseases are also not as straightforward nor as easily diagnosed as getting an infection. Someone may have cardiovascular disease or neurodegeneration already in the fold, but it is difficult to diagnose in the early stages where it could be possibly treated better, or its course slowed down.

It is very important to understand how many times you do not stop to think and analyze the effects that your actions cause on your body, like what the food you eat does to you or what your persistent thought patterns do in the end. What about the work you have or all the responsibilities at home? Are you stressing a lot about losing your spouse and being alone? Do you feel rushed and short on time? All these and more can turn on the alarm of stress that you must learn to turn off. It cannot be on all the time.

If you do not turn off stress, it can produce effects down the road. Even though you do not see the disease, it does not mean it does not exist. It is just that it has not manifested physically, and thus diagnosing it is difficult.

To live free of the fear of a painful aging process or early death, you must learn to care for your entire multidimensional being by eating better, exercising the right way, getting more quality sleep, breathing better, being more mindful and present, taking the right supplements, cultivating better habits and ethics that purify your body, mind, and spirit, etc.

The goal of this chapter was not to be overly negative about the effects of stress, but to educate you because it is very important to know the effects stress can have on your body and later what you can do to minimize or eliminate these risks altogether. Stress management is not just about peace and rejuvenation, but about your health and wellness as well. Let's continue with food or body stress.

Chapter 4:

Healing your Temple

*"Your body is your temple. Keep it pure and clean
for the soul to reside in."*

— B.K.S. Iyengar

For you to be successful long-term in this or any other program or venture, your body must remain free of disease, retain its strength and vitality, and possess higher levels of energy to sustain deeper practices conducive to Self-Realization or, at the bare minimum, higher awareness and stability. However, due to excesses, poor habits or diet, or lack of proper exercise, our body is just not fit for long periods of study, introspection, exercise, or concentration.

Furthermore, if you want to establish a healthy routine in the early morning before work, which is ideal, you must have the energy and resolve to do so. However, this will be difficult if your body is stressed and inflamed and is a source of distraction, pain, and suffering.

How can we expect to make meaningful progress toward mental and physical health, when we are a nutrient- and sleep-deprived culture? Physiologically speaking, our brain and other systems are just not well balanced and likely do not produce a healthy profile of neurochemicals, hormones, gene expression, cell signaling, etc. We only exacerbate the problem when we consume phytonutrient poor, energy dense, and toxic foods.

If you do not take care of your body, then how can you expect to enjoy freedom from chronic illnesses, aging, and even common acute disease like a cold or the flu? You can become relatively free from any physical ailment if you live, eat, and breathe in a healthier and more powerful way.

To master the art of living, you must transcend your bodily limitations, which you impose on yourself due to your own habits, conditions, preconceptions, and behaviors. Your body is where your consciousness, who you are, resides. Thus, honor it and purify it with the right food, stimuli, thoughts, speech, and action.

As with any of the suggestions given in this book, taking care of yourself should be one of many adjunct therapies you include in your daily activities. For a person who is very dedicated and masters the art of living, many benefits will ensue, including avoiding any or most diseases, lustrous complexion, radiant health, increased vitality and power, and slower aging process.

These changes can of course have a useful effect on the rest of the practices outlined in this book. Think of all the times you have been sick, injured, or in pain. How much can you do for yourself or others when you have the flu or are dealing with some chronic ailment that limits your expression? Even if you find yourself already struggling with limitations or a chronic condition, changing your approach to health will yield wonderful results.

Although I will emphasize the need for a better diet with intake of mainly *sattvic*[27] (whole plant-based) food, healing herbs, and superfoods, ingestion is more than just what goes through your mouth. You must also consider other sources of ingestion, including through your senses. For example, you take in subtle elements when you read, watch the news, or listen to music. The type of stimuli you expose your body – and more importantly, your mind – to matters and can have significant effects on your level of wellness, tranquility, health.

These subtle energy aspects of health are acting constantly, and I will touch upon them in Chapter 11. In this chapter, I will emphasize the more physical aspects of health that we often do not consider. It will encompass over two decades of work, research, and my own experimentation of the right combination of foods, supplements, and herbs, with a focus on reducing stress and inflammation. For those interested in a more individual program for your constitution, personality, and body type, please visit me at ramasrootedtree.com or on social media.

Mindful Eating

Mindful eating is a wonderful practice that can help you to rediscover a healthy relationship with food and avoid mindless eating that can lead to overeating and less enjoyment of what you eat. During mindful, eating you bring full awareness of what you are experiencing while eating and drinking. What do you feel in your mouth or as the food goes down to your stomach? How does your energy level change? You should observe the food very closely, taking your time to savor it to enjoy its rich textures and flavors.

During mindful eating, you become much more sensitive to the inner workings of your body and to the thought processes that may arise before, during, and after the meal. What is going on in your mind as you eat? Did your mood influence the decision to start eating, or maybe you felt anxious and decided to grab a snack to distract you?

You will notice that your mind will be pulled away from what you eat or drink. You may feel the urge to grab your phone to make a call or search for something on the internet, turn on the television, or grab a book to read. Resist these urges to replace the attention on the food with something else and just go back to concentrating on the eating process. It will be difficult at first, but the benefits are worth it. Thus, start simple and make slow changes in your eating habits to bring greater awareness and appreciation to this process. Mindful eating can help you to reclaim the freedom with eating you enjoyed as a child. Try this practice with my favorite fruit for mindful eating, the pomegranate (Appendix B).

Try doing this practice while at work at least once a week. Find a quiet place to eat in silence. If you have an office, close the door and eat quietly, or go to the car and sit by yourself to eat. You can even do some breathing exercises in those scenarios prior to eating or at some other point for a quick mindful break. It could even be something as simple as sipping your tea or coffee with full awareness and concentration.

Integrate this with your family by asking everyone to eat in silence for a few minutes. They can also try to eat mindfully and think about what was involved in getting this food to the table. The sunlight within it, the indiscriminate rain that gave rise to it, the farmers who tirelessly worked the land, the driver who brought it to the local supermarket, the person who prepared the meal, etc. They should give thanks to all the sources that helped provide this food to them before resuming normal eating. This is an excellent practice to do with children.

Ahimsa and Diet

To bring exceptional tranquility and peace into your life, you must integrate one of the most important ethical concepts of yoga that Gandhi embodied so beautifully, *ahimsa,* or non-violence. Your actions, either directly or indirectly, should not cause harm to another living organism or to the environment, and thus yoga espouses a diet that is free from harm.

This harm is not just that you eat meat, for example, and that it harms cows and also leads to environmental destruction, but more importantly for the purposes of this book, that you are harming yourself by eating toxic, dead animal food, or overcooked and fried food that contributes to chronic illnesses, accelerated aging, and cognitive impairment in the long run. Treat your body as a temple for your spirit and feed it the right combination of both gross (i.e., solid food) and subtle elements (i.e., sensory impressions).

To achieve perfect expression of *ahimsa* is not the intention of this book and can be quite challenging to do for most. However, what you can do is to get educated and make smarter choices to reduce the chances of getting one or more of the chronic diseases that stress exacerbates. These include cardiovascular disease, diabetes, cancer, inflammation, etc.

By switching your diet more toward a whole plant-based one, you will drastically improve your health and can often reverse the effects of many chronic ailments (i.e., lower your cholesterol and blood sugar, lose weight, etc.). Ideally, you should consider adopting a vegetarian or vegan diet, but if this is too difficult or you just do not want to make such a lifestyle change, then increase your intake of many of the foods described below and in Appendix B. By doing so, you live more ethically responsibly, reduce inflammation and toxicity in your body, and can have the health that you deserve, thereby freeing you in large part from disease.

Stress-related chronic diseases and inflammation are caused by diets rich in animal-products.[28] Red meat and pork are the worst in this regard. Raw foods, like salads, cruciferous vegetables, dark greens, and rich colorful fruits help to detoxify the body and increase your subtle energy reserve for better aging and disease prevention. These foods are some of the highest scoring foods when it comes to enhancing mental health (i.e., depression) as they contain many important vitamins, minerals, and omega-3 fatty acids (EPA and DHA).[29]

In addition, these healthy options are phytonutrient-dense and balanced with the right amount of protein, unsaturated fats, vitamins, minerals, and energy. Avoid nutrient-poor food high in calories, saturated fat, and preservatives, such canned or processed foods. Eat organic, especially from local farmer's markets, to support local community, enhance nutrient content, and minimize exposure to chemical fertilizers and sprays that contain harmful and sometimes cancer-causing chemicals.[30,31,32]

If you build up your cells, tissues, and organs with unhealthy and toxic food or other substances (i.e., alcohol or drugs), your body will then be diseased, damaged, or deficient. A diseased, damaged, or deficient body will reflect the same deficiencies and problems onto the mind because the physical body is the substrate or grossest manifestation of the mind.

Therefore, eat foods that sustain the natural state of your body and build it with all the right components and with little to no toxicity. For the purposes of this book, consider a diet that nurtures your nervous system, in particular, (i.e., omega fatty acids, nutrient-dense, antioxidant, and anti-inflammatory). In this way you can develop *ojas* or vitality and power for your body and mind.

Foods that Cause or Eliminate Inflammation

In the previous chapter, I mentioned how most diseases involve activation of stress pathways. Like chronic stress, chronic inflammation is also a key component of chronic Western illnesses. Interestingly, excessive inflammation plays a significant role in the progression and/or onset of stress related diseases, which suggests a common pathway linking them both.

In addition, stress can increase systemic inflammatory responses through stress hormones. Not surprisingly, inflammation is linked to many of the diseases discussed in the previous chapter, including depression, neurodegenerative diseases, cancer, diabetes, and cardiovascular disease.[33]

Therefore, avoiding foods that induce inflammation in the body becomes crucial. In table below, I list foods that cause inflammation and those that eliminate it. Notice how it supports what I mentioned in the previous section on *ahimsa*.

The more you increase what eliminates inflammation, the better you will feel, the less stressed your body will be, and the more energy you will have, since you are not fighting toxicity and inflammation as often. Numerous studies not cited here have linked inflammatory processes to depression, possibly due to the ability of inflammatory cytokines preventing the conversion of tryptophan to serotonin. Furthermore, reducing inflammation may decrease neuronal loss and increased risk of neurodegenerative conditions, like Alzheimer's disease. Increasing omega-3 fatty acids, found mainly in plant sources, may help protect the brain and benefit your mental health (i.e., anxiety).[34]

Eliminates Inflammation	Nuts (Especially Raw)	Avocado	Dark Leafy Greens	Tart Cherries	Orange Fruits & Vegetables	Olive & Coconut Oil	Pineapple	Turmeric Ginger Garlic
Causes Inflammation	Gluten	Casein (Found in Dairy)	Fried Foods	Processed Meats	Meat & Dairy	Safflower, Sunflower, Soy, Corn Oils	Corn Syrup & Soft Drinks	Fast Foods

Healing Herbs & Supplements

The herbs or supplements listed in this chapter are included here due to their strong adaptogenic effects. An adaptogen is a natural substance capable of promoting balance and reducing stress and inflammation. I have included additional dietary suggestions in Appendix A to leave few stones unturned when it comes to enhancing your health and well-being.

Holy Basil, or tulsi, is an herb used for thousands of years not only for cooking, but also as an adjunct treatment for coughs, colds, and the flu, as it helps to cleanse the respiratory tract of toxins. This holistic healing tonic has many uses, but the one most relevant to this book is its ability to act as an adaptogen.

Holy basil increases endurance and enhances metabolism in animals. It is also able, though it is unknown how, to reduce the stress response in stressful environments in both animals and humans. Holy basil has anti-depressant and anti-anxiety effects, similar to drugs commonly prescribed to patients.[35,36]

Basil contains a compound called eugenol, which is a natural antioxidant. *In vitro* and *in vivo* experiments show that this compound can block oxidative damage from free radicals five times more effectively than vitamin E, a powerful antioxidant in its own right.[37]

Other uses of holy basil include: (1) detoxing due to its high antioxidants counts, (2) wound healing when used as an extract, (3) lowering weight, blood sugar, and cholesterol, (4) improving symptoms of stress-induced ulcers, and (5) reducing inflammation.[38,39]

Tulsi should be taken as a tea using leaves, but can also be used in cooking, in salads, and in smoothies. Eugenol-rich tulsi extract liquid capsules are another option for daily consumption. In foods, basil leaves offer a rich aroma that enhances many different meals.

Ashwagandha, or Indian ginseng, is another ancient medicine and, as one of the most important Ayurvedic herbs, it is used traditionally to counter stress by reducing cortisol levels,[40,41] increasing energy levels, and enhancing brain function,[42,43] all of which are relevant to the main topics of this book. With its high concentration of withanolides,[44] ashwagandha helps to fight inflammation and tumor growth.[45]

Due to its many benefits, ashwagandha has become a very popular supplement. These other benefits include amongst many others: (1) increasing insulin secretion to help reduce blood sugar levels,[46,47] (2) slowing the growth and spread of tumor cells,[48,49] and (3) reducing anxiety.[50,51]

In general, you can take ashwagandha in capsule form of ground root (two capsules depending on dosage, once daily).

Turmeric (or its active ingredient curcumin) is another in an increasing line of medicinal spices and herbs. Its benefits are extensive, and I cannot list all the great effects this root, especially curcumin, has to offer your health. Due to the myriad benefits it offers to human health, I, in fact, take it daily, whether it is in capsule or soft gel form, or as a fresh, peeled root in a smoothie, or juiced.

I encourage others, especially athletes or anyone with joint inflammation, to take it daily as well. Turmeric has powerful anti-inflammatory effects and is a very strong antioxidant, but its effects are enhanced when taking extracts containing higher amounts of tetra-hydro curcuminoids.[52] Due to the poor absorption of curcumin, it helps to take the supplement with black pepper, which contains piperine that increases the absorption of curcumin.[53] More recent versions have enhanced its bioavailability (absorption) and benefits by formulating it with black cumin oil, since curcumin is fat soluble.

Curcumin is such a powerful anti-inflammatory that its effects match anti-inflammatory drugs, with no side effects.[54,55] It is also a very powerful antioxidant that neutralizes free radicals[56,57] and enhances the function of your body's own antioxidant enzymes.[58,59]

Additional benefits of curcumin include but are not limited to: (1) treating arthritis,[60] (2) anti-aging,[61] (3) an adjunct therapy for depression, possibly by boosting dopamine and serotonin levels,[62,63,64] and (4) cancer prevention and maybe even treatment.[65]

Ayurvedic formulations: Chyawanprash and Amrit Kalash are described in Ayurvedic texts as having a wide range of benefits, as they contain a number of nutritive and healing herbs. These are typically taken in a mixture of herbs and ghee, and thus are not vegan. However, as a person who eats vegan, I make the exception for these two *rasayanas* that are of immense value to our well-being. *Rasayana* is a rejuvenating treatment for all tissues of the body that enhances longevity, health, and well-being.

Chyawanprash is taken in one to two teaspoon doses every day, usually in the morning. Studies involving chyawanprash are lacking, other than a few studies I found on its immunostimulatory and anti-aging skin effects. Nonetheless, its key ingredient, called amlaki or amla, has been studied more. Amlaki is renowned for its rich antioxidant content, especially vitamin C, which is preserved throughout the preparation thanks to the presence of tannins.[66] Whether it does what it is reported to do is still up for debate, but chyawanprash is nonetheless a staple of my daily diet and is very nourishing, rejuvenating, and allopathic. Therefore, as it supports healthy aging, promotes systemic well-being, and enhances vitality, chyawanprash is a true elixir of life.

Amrit Kalash is a nectar of immortality as its name implies (*amrit* = immortality and *kalash* = pot or pitcher). In essence, it is a pot filled with immortality or longevity. Amrit Kalash is a mixture of a number of different plants and herbs, some of which are rare and precious, and which promote perfect health and longevity.

Amrit Kalash comes as a nectar (paste) and as ambrosia (tablet). Both should be consumed for better results. The nectar is taken first (one and a half teaspoons) and the tablet thirty minutes later. Indeed, as of the writing of this book, I have been taking Amrit Kalash nectar and ambrosia for at least two years, and I have yet to get sick at all. Whether that is just a coincidence or due to the myriad of other wellness practices my body enjoys can be argued, but nonetheless highly positive results are there and are supported by scientific studies.

Just like chyawanprash, by containing an ideal mix of ingredients using refined and ancient, advanced knowledge, these *rasayanas* promote balance and thus help to reduce stress and inflammation in the body. In addition, Amrit Kalash prevents the deterioration of the immune system as you age, thus keeping us healthier.[67] It may also help inhibit the formation of cancer cells by enhancing immune function[68,69] and help rejuvenate an aging nervous system by increasing the activities of antioxidant enzymes.[70]

Diindolmethane (DIM) is the principal breakdown product of indole 3-carbinol, which is a chemical found in what are arguably the healthiest of all vegetables, the cruciferous vegetables (such as broccoli, kale, brussels sprouts, collards, etc.). Consumption of these vegetables is essential to our health and numerous studies support the role of DIM as an anti-cancer agent. It also boasts anti-aging effects, as it helps to balance levels of hormones known to decrease as you age (i.e., estrogen and testosterone), which enhance energy, mood, and libido in both men and women.

Even though DIM is sold as a supplement, I would suggest first increasing your intake of whole plant-based food high in cruciferous vegetables, such as kale and broccoli, which offer a number of benefits from anti-cancer agents like sulforaphane;[71] flavonoids like Quercetin and Kaempferol with strong anti-inflammatory, antioxidant, and anti-cancer effects;[72] minerals and other key vitamins; and beta carotene. These vegetables are a true gift to humans and should be a significant part of everyone's diet.

Triphala is another staple of Ayurvedic medicine and consists of three key medicinal plants. Firstly, amla, or Indian gooseberry, which is a very nutritious fruit that has been shown to inhibit cancer growth.[73,74] It also contains powerful phytochemicals like tannins, curcuminoids, etc.[75]

The second ingredient is bibhitaki, which contains many powerful phytochemicals, similar to amlaki.[76] An animal-based diet high in beef and/or pork can cause a buildup of uric acid in our bodies, especially our joints, contributing to arthritis as we age. Bibhitaki reduces uric acid levels, demonstrating anti-inflammatory capabilities.[77]

Lastly, triphala contains haritaki, the king of medicines in Ayurveda, which possesses powerful phytochemicals like terpenes and polyphenols. Due to this, haritaki has been shown to possess strong anti-inflammatory and antioxidant properties. Therefore, the combination of all three is a prized herbal formulation for treating arthritis and protecting against cancer.

Maca is another of the great cruciferous vegetables that I mentioned earlier that are so valuable to our health. This adaptogen helps to combat stress and fatigue and is very nutritious, as it is high in protein, iron, and vitamin C. As with the other holistic plants you saw previously, maca has many powerful bioactive compounds, such as flavonoids. Maca has been reported to increase fertility in men, relieve menopause symptoms,[78] enhance energy and sports endurance,[79] increase libido,[80,81] promote balance, and improve mood by reducing anxiety and symptoms of depression.[82,83] In addition, maca prevents age-related cognitive decline.[84] Lastly, due to its high polyphenolic compounds, maca may prevent memory impairments. Take maca as ground root powder in fresh juices or smoothies or as tablets or capsules. With its nutty flavor, maca pairs well with cacao, which I discuss in Appendix A.

Matcha is a green tea rich in catechins, powerful antioxidants. Different from regular green tea, matcha contains up to 137 times the catechins,[85] which can reduce cell damage, inflammation, and risk of chronic diseases.[86] Matcha can also enhance brain function, including attention and memory[87] and may decrease stress levels and enhance relaxation.[88] Because it contains so many healthy compounds, matcha may prevent cancer.[89] In particular, one of its catechins, epigallocatechin-3-gallate (EGCG), helps to fight off a number of different cancers. EGCG can also block the production of molecules that cause joint damage in patients.[90] Matcha powder is very easy to prepare as a tea or to add to smoothies and even baked goods.

Magnesium: Diets low in magnesium correlate with increased anxiety and stress. Furthermore, magnesium supplementation may attenuate anxiety symptoms.[91] Interestingly, magnesium increases the levels of neurotransmitter GABA, which is a target signaling molecule for reducing anxiety and improving sleep. By modulating the HPA axis, magnesium is a central player of the stress response system of our bodies. Therefore, diets rich in magnesium or intake of magnesium drinks can help a person feel calmer. Foods rich in magnesium include leafy greens, spinach, whole grains, nuts, legumes, seeds, tofu, avocado, bananas, dragon fruit, sweet potatoes, and even one of my favorite treats, dark chocolate. Note: Zinc may also be another key metal that shows similar links with depression[92] and anxiety[93] in animal studies and improves the clinical effects of antidepressants.[94]

Now the questions I am often asked are: How do I integrate all of these herbs or supplements into my diet? Do I have to integrate them all? Firstly, no you do not have to integrate them all into your diet and certainly not all in one day. However, many can be integrated into your diet as you try to consume as many of these superfoods and herbs as often as possible. Capsule or dry forms should only be an option if you cannot get the fresh or whole version. There are a few I do consume daily, like triphala, Amrit Kalash, and chyawanprash (alternate taking these two, if too expensive to consume both daily), turmeric with curcumin, and matcha green tea, amongst a few others, but most I consume regularly, especially in smoothies, juices, or cereals and salads.

A balanced diet high in whole plant-based foods, nuts, seeds, roots, legumes, grains is what you are meant to eat and what is best for your physical and mental health. This diet is real preventative medicine that keeps your entire body in optimal condition by helping to maintain ideal levels of key molecules in the body, especially the brain, as I emphasize in this book (see Appendix A as well). Moreover, a whole plant-based diet does not contribute to cardiovascular disease, inflammation, and other chronic ailments, but in fact prevents them altogether because of the powerful, healing phytochemicals it contains. These fresh, unprocessed, live, and whole plant-based foods illustrate the axiom, "let food be thy medicine," very clearly.

The high antioxidant content in these healing foods and herbs makes them potential candidates in the treatment of depression and anxiety.[95] Not only that, but these foods reduce activation of stress pathways in our bodies and may prevent or ameliorate a number of chronic Western ailments. For information on additional superfoods please go to Appendix B.

For recipes and additional health and dietary tips, please visit me on social media or ramasrootedtree.com.

Healing Mantras

The practice of mantra can be a wonderful adjunct remedy for healing our consciousness and creating an inner resonance of power, vitality, and focus. Mantras are great in that they can be practiced anywhere, whether you want to infuse your *pranayama* (concentrated breathing) practice, while driving or walking, in the shower, or even while lying in bed. Ideally, a mantra should be given by someone who has brought the mantra to life and considers it ideal for your development. Despite this, I will recommend a few mantras of general or healing nature. If you would like to hear a recording of any mantra, including the ones in this book, or if you would like more mantra suggestions, please visit ramasrootedtree.com.

Om Apadamapa Hataram Dataram Sarva Sampadam
Loka Bhi Raman Sri Raman Bhuyo Bhuyo Namam-yaham
"Om, O most compassionate Rama! Please send your healing energy right here to the Earth, to the Earth. Salutations."

Rama represents a role model of *ahimsa* and living with the highest of ethics and standards. He blessed and healed many in his lifetime in part due to being able to make things so just by speaking it, as a number of sages in the past have been able to do. The healing potencies of his name are amongst the most powerful even for a skeptic. The mantra above may have one of the most powerful healing effects as it stimulates the awakening of dormant energy in the solar plexus region, thanks to the seed sound Ram. Thomas Ashley-Farrand describes this mantra healing various individuals with different physical or mental conditions.[96]

Om Trayumbakam Yajamahe Sughandhim Pushti Vardanam
Urvarukamiva Bandhanan Mrityor Muksheeya Mamritat
"Shelter me, O three-eyed Lord Shiva. Bless me with health and immortality and sever me from the clutches of death, even as a cucumber is cut from its creeper."

The *Markandeya* or *Mahamrityunjaya* mantra is named after a legendary boy named Markandeya that was saved from death by Shiva just before his sixteenth birthday. The mantra contains immense healing potential and can slow the aging process if practiced sufficiently and correctly. Thomas Ashley-Farrand describes this mantra healing viral infections, maybe in part due to an immune boosting effect.[97]

You can repeat any mantra at least 108 times or a multiple of that number. To keep track of the count, you can use a meditation necklace with 108 beads. Hold the first bead with your thumb and index finger and slide from one bead to the next after every repetition (internally or aloud). If you cannot practice this many repetitions, then fit in as many as you can.

Note: Any mantra in this book is universal in nature, despite containing anthropomorphized principles such as Rama, Shiva, or later on Ganesha. No matter what tradition or spiritual path you choose, you can supplement the practices in this book with any recitation described and many others not included. These will increase your concentration and spiritual development.

Mantras can be practiced at any time. You can concentrate on or repeat the mantra mentally while doing some of the breathing techniques described in the next chapter or during meditation. They can also be chanted out loud and I can email you files with any mantra recording, if you register on my website and request a recording to practice at home on your own. Mantras are also excellent to help disrupt the activities of the monkey mind described in Chapter 11, when you find your mind inundated with a constant stream of thoughts, which could exacerbate anxiety, worry, or stress.

Mantras can be enjoyed with music as well and in a community setting with others to build collective energy and power. For example, you can enjoy listening and chanting along with kirtan music, which is very popular across the world and specifically in yoga studios and retreats.

The Story of Katherine

Katherine was thirty-eight years old when came to me. She was about fifty pounds overweight. She was married and had a seven-year-old child.

She worked full-time in a corporate job. She had responsibilities at her job that often contributed to her feelings of anxiety. However, her biggest stress trigger was that she was overweight, and this was causing her to be very depressed and hopeless. She desired to be attractive to others and to feel more comfortable and confident in her body.

Before her son was born, Katherine battled with weight control but was always able to get her weight to her desired target through fad diets. However, after her son, no matter what she ate or what diet she kept she simply could not lose the weight. In fact, she was gaining weight, a little every year to the point where she had now developed chronic conditions usually associated with older people. She had hypertension, high cholesterol, and was even in the beginning stages of type-2 diabetes.

She was frustrated with herself and her body, leaving her depressed with how she looked. This began to affect her outside of the house as her confidence and self-esteem dwindled. Between her weight, her job, and taking care of her son and husband, she was always tired.

Katherine tried to eat healthy but sometimes she would eat very late in the evening when her metabolism was slower. At other times, she was so frustrated that she would not eat at all. Sometimes, she was so depressed that all she did was eat...and on these days, she ate all the junk food that she could find. Somehow, this made her feel better while she was eating it but later it made her feel horrible about herself.

She rarely wanted to go out, never wanted to dress up, or dressed to hide her body, and was never encouraged enough to wear an ounce of lipstick. Honestly, there were days she left the house without brushing her hair. Katherine will tell you herself that she felt like she had hit the end of her life.

There were days that she did not want to get out of her bed. Although her husband was supportive, she struggled with internal feelings of guilt because she knew that at the end of the day, she was not there one hundred percent for him or for her son. Katherine was so stressed about her weight and her inability to lose it that it dampened her personality and pizzazz. She thought longingly of the past when she was younger and possessed more confidence and self-esteem.

I met Katherine at a family event. She was friends with a colleague of my wife, Norma. I could immediately see the burdens she was carrying. The external obstacles she had fixated her mind onto were keeping her spirit caged and oppressed. She was not seeing what I could see through all the barriers: that she was a beautiful, vibrant spirit that had just lost her passion and love for life and was lacking direction and focus.

I approached Katherine and just started talking to her without any self-interest or expectation. I wanted her to feel wanted, special, and heard. I wanted her to know that she did matter and that there were options to help her that she had not considered up until then.

As she opened up, I just listened. I could feel her pain and her insecurities. With tears in her eyes and mine, I embraced her and told her: "This is not a coincidence. I am here for a reason. Please give me the opportunity to work with you. I know I can help reverse most, if not all, of what you are going through, both physically and mentally." She agreed to an initial consultation and thus we scheduled a time for the following week.

During that initial phone call, I started by saying: "Kathy, if this is going to work, I need you to have faith in me and remain open and receptive to all that I have to offer. My heart is open and ready to give. Can you be the perfect receptacle and student? Can you do all I ask of you? It will not be easy, but I know you can do this, and I will be there as long as you want and need me to be."

An awkward silence ensued and for a moment there, I thought she had put up her walls again and I had lost her. However, to my surprise she burst out crying and replied, "Thank you, Dr. Ramos. I have not felt accepted by anyone other than my husband and child in a long time. I want to overcome this, but I have struggled to find the right solution. I feel stuck and tired. I am committed to doing whatever you ask of me. I need your help!"

Over the course of the next eight weeks, I worked to teach her the program described in this book. I would visit her at her home, and we would sometimes talk over the phone or via Zoom or FaceTime. I designed a food plan to transition her into a diet heavier on whole plants, superfoods, supplements, and healing herbs, many of which I describe in this book. I gave her recipes to follow and a plan of what to eat and snack on and when. Within a matter of just two weeks, her blood sugar and cholesterol levels had dropped significantly to the point that they were within normal range. Even her blood pressure had improved and would improve further as she learned how to engage her autonomic nervous system with precision and care using yogic techniques. Her body's inflammatory and stress responses lessened to the point that she actually felt different, as if her body were no longer screaming out in pain, and thus her mind could rest more easily and devote more time to healing herself.

In addition, I started teaching a number of self-care practices. I wanted her to rediscover the love for herself that she had lost. Who she was had been there all along, but the exterior, including her body, had changed. Her experiences had taken a hold of her and she became disconnected, like most of us, to her True Self.

Therefore, once she had learned many of the techniques and practices, I wanted her to integrate, she decided to work with me for the next twelve months to implement these changes and to receive therapeutic yoga sessions on a weekly basis. During this year, she deepened her meditative practice with my guidance to see that she was more than just her body, brain, and mind. She could let go of the notion that she was an idea that she did not like, but instead was vast, free, and grand. She learned to relax, let go, and just be.

As she lost weight and increased her energy level, she was more able to undertake a formal yoga *asana* practice and even joined a local yoga studio. She felt better, stronger, and more confident. I could see a fire in her eyes that had not been there before. She had determination and vision to take this further now on her own.

I am deeply touched by Katherine, as I am with all my clients, who never cease to amaze me by showing the power of human resolve. With willpower, she overcame her self-imposed limitations to see herself as a free spirit full of creativity, health, and power. Slowly, she was able to let go of the blame she would have often affixed to the exterior for her problems. Her body was no longer the limiting factor in her life.

Her mind, now an asset, empowered her to do more and be more than she could have ever imagined. She realized that she had it all within herself, but she needed help finding it. Once she had found a higher self, independent of all the barriers she had put up, she was able to assert herself, live with greater passion, free of fear and worry. With confidence, she no longer struggled with bouts of depression. Happiness reigned supreme in her heart and in her life. When in doubt I can look back at a photo of Katherine, and I look at her bright eyes and tender smile and know that all the work and effort is worth it. With her health in hand, she was able to pursue the transpersonal growth she had been longing for all along.

Chapter 5:

Friend or Foe?

"*The greatest weapon against stress is our ability to choose one thought over another.*"
— William James

Tao of Stress

In Chapter 3, you saw how the SNS was able to activate the stress response. This does not mean, however, that stress or SNS are to be viewed negatively. There are moments in our life when you need to augment the activity of the SNS, and at other times, you need to be able to diminish its activities. These opposing dynamic forces are at the heart of helping to maintain balance when faced with stress (allostasis), keep your nervous and endocrine systems tuned, and promote better health and wellness.

Even if your PNS, with its so-called beneficial effects of relaxation and rejuvenation, were overly active compared to the SNS, you would struggle with depression, lethargy, or with very little energy and motivation to do anything. On the other hand, if your SNS were running awry, you would

51

be very anxious, suffer from insomnia, react with anger or aggression, and have lower attentive capabilities and reasoning skills. Therefore, the problem is not that stress is something negative. The key is to have physical, emotional, and mental balance.

You have the power to influence that balance point depending on the mechanisms you choose to use to deal with unavoidable stresses you will encounter in life. You can consciously control the degree of stress you are experiencing by identifying the events or people that increase stress and changing the perspective you take toward them. You have more control than you think. Change the way you see yourself in relation to these stressors.

Enhance the resources available to you, so that you can have more energy, a clearer perspective, a sharper mind, and a calmer disposition to deal with stressful situations. Thus, work toward enhancing your psychological and physical well-being through meditation, higher ethical standards, improved diet, and yogic exercises, described throughout the book and found on my website, ramasrootedtree.com.

You must find a balance point in your life to stop amplifying stress to the extent that you do and pushing the limits of your body and mind beyond what is comfortable and healthy. You are a being that needs to live in balance for overall health, wellness, and peace of mind.

The body has natural mechanisms to reestablish this balance. For example, when the body temperature goes above a set point, the body will initiate a response to cool itself down by dilating peripheral blood vessels and diverting warm blood to the surface of the skin where heat can evaporate sweat, lowering your body temperature as hotter water molecules move away from the body. If the body produces a hormone, it will not keep making more endlessly. Once cells have made enough hormone, the body does not want to keep making more, and thus will turn on signaling pathways within cells to decrease its production and release.

Therefore, the body or the cells that make it up can increase the levels of a substance when it needs it and decrease it when it does not. In the same way, when am stressed, I increase SNS activation, but when

I am not, I decrease SNS activation and increase PNS activation to reestablish balance.

If you are constantly under extended periods of intermittent stress, your body will be unable to reestablish balance, which, as I described in Chapter 3, leads to a number of health concerns. You have to find a way to balance the activities of the SNS and PNS. Living with the accelerator pressed on in the background all the time is not what you were designed to do. If you do, you will suffer the consequences in the long run.

You need to find way to build tranquility and calmness in your body with the neutralizing effect of the PNS. Finding a way out of the vicious cycle of doing, if even for ten to fifteen minutes, can provide you with great benefits. Mastering the art of just being and enjoying the simple fact that you are alive and can breathe can be extremely valuable for your mental health and overall well-being. In the next chapter, I will share some techniques to reestablish this balance and reduce unwanted tension in the body. These techniques involve activation of the PNS, reducing SNS activation, or harmonizing the two using your breath and concentration.

The breath can be a very powerful tool for relaxation, as a recent study in a premier journal, *Science*, showed. The results of this recent study suggest that deep, concentrated breathing reduces the activity of a key brainstem nucleus called the locus coeruleus that projects to the PFC. This reduction induces a calming effect and boosts attentional capabilities by enhancing PFC functioning. In Chapter 3, we talked about the inverted U of the stress response. Well, slow, controlled breathing shifts the inverted U (in this case of norepinephrine) to the left and restores optimal PFC functioning.[98] Thus, learning how to breathe more effectively is a key to conquering stress and achieving balance.

Stress and DNA Dynamics

You often forget you possess a biological self that is your body. This body is made up of cells and these cells contain genetic material called DNA (short for deoxyribonucleic acid). Our DNA, as many of us know, contains our genes, and these genes (genotype) are responsible for permitting the cells to make proteins, the "machines" or "workers" of the cell that produce our traits. Proteins are the ones that carry out reactions in our cells and that help to produce the physical manifestation (phenotype) that you see. This is an oversimplification, but nonetheless will suffice to illustrate the point I am about to make.

There is a concept that people often have, which is that "I am born with a certain genetic makeup and that in a way my genes heavily dictate my fate." What most do not know, unless they have studied biology or physiology, is that our genes, more appropriately our gene expression, are dynamic, and change depending on our experiences. As you saw in Chapter 3, chronic stress is one of those experiences that changes the pattern of gene expression, and thus the proteins available, in ways that are detrimental to our health.

Remember that positive and enriching experiences also change our gene expression in ways that are beneficial to our cells and body. Therefore, you should enhance these types of experiences in your life and reduce chronic stress and negative experiences, habits, or behaviors. While chronic stress leads to neuronal atrophy, enrichment enhances neuronal complexity and connectivity. This is entirely due to adaptive, genetic, and biochemical changes that modify our dynamic and plastic cells.

Do not look at symptoms as something negative. I do not want you to feel burdened by the thought: "What have I done to myself?" Where you are right now does not matter as much as what you do from this point on. You can start changing what you have already projected onto your body by reprogramming your cells starting with your DNA and its gene expression.

As you will see later in Chapter 9, living in the past is not productive. Instead, focus all your energies on the present to get past your limitations and find greater health, happiness, and peace. Look at your current symptoms as information that is telling you a lot about how unbalanced your body, mind, or spirit are. You can change, like a radio player, your frequency to tune into a higher frequency and a healthier and more powerful wavelength to play a different melody with the strings of your DNA and its associated genes.

A stressor is anything that takes you away from homeostatic balance. Under crisis or eminent death, stress hormones can reestablish the acutely lost homeostasis or preserve the body from injury or even death. Often, however, you are not out of balance, but you anticipate that you will be due to a variety of events or people that you perceive as stressful.

In those moments that you perceive a situation like that, especially if it happens often, someone may describe you as neurotic, anxious, or paranoid. Unlike an animal who turns on the stress response for acute bursts to survive (antelope in the savannah getting chased by a lion), you turn it on for psychological reasons (i.e., how do I pay my mortgage?).

The stress response did not evolve for that reason, and its chronic activation can have disastrous consequences long-term for our health. Learning to control our thoughts, memories, and emotions to life's circumstances is thus key to avoiding turning on this system inappropriately and in a way that can harm us and our loved ones. In Chapter 3, I described how there is an inverted U response where too much or too little is not ideal. What you need is an optimal level of stimulation and activation. Too much and you can begin to feel stressed, anxious, neurotic, or sick.

Oddly, although animals do not normally self-induce psychological stress, scientists put animals like rats in stressful situations that induce psychological stress, and then examine changes within cells and organ structures like the brain. For example, Hans Selye, one of the pioneers of stress research, showed stress-induced ulcers in rats. Later studies showed links between stress and many other diseases as well (Chapter 3) and on recovery from illness or surgery. One of the landmark results in this field is that stress changes your gene expression, as I have emphasized before.

Remember that stress in the short-term can be a good thing by giving you increased energy and power during moments of survival or imminent danger. The problems begin when this state of hyperarousal becomes permanent without actually dealing with or overcoming your stressors. This can increase your stress levels, along with associated neurochemicals and hormones, leading to feelings of hopelessness and helplessness due to depletion of nervous resources. The key is to stop reacting to stress and begin to respond to it with measure, poise, and control.

External Support vs. Internal Regulators

The stress pathway is modulated by appraisal, perception, and evaluation, meaning that if you do not perceive stress to be uncontrollable or you do not even recognize or ignore it, it will not have a significant effect on your body.

You could have two people in the same room, exposed to the same stressor, for the same amount of time, and one person will show a physiological response and the other one will not. In addition, if you feel like you have an escape or a refuge (i.e., the arms of a parent or spouse or an empathetic and supporting friend or boss) the effects of stress can be neutralized.

Having support matters. You do not have to do this alone and should not have to. If you do not have that support or do not know how to integrate these changes, then get it from an experienced spiritual teacher or guru, a therapist, or a coach. The support of your family is also crucial. Nurture the connections within your family circle to create a collective consciousness, a single organism with greater energy reserves to deal with life's unexpected turns, trials, and tribulations.

Studies show that modulators of stress, like an outlet (exercise), a distractor, social support, or a drug have only modest effects. What truly has a more powerful effect are internal regulators, mainly a sense of control. For example, exposure of a group of animals to stress causes significant changes in nervous system gene expression not seen in the control, unstressed animals. Moreover, when you compare both groups, there are clear differences in the proteins being expressed and their effects on the body.[99,100] Therefore, even if you stress two animals for the same amount of time, but only one can control or escape the stressor (i.e., an animal presses a lever to stop stressful stimuli), then only the one without the control lever demonstrates the elevated physiological stress parameters.[101]

These results are very interesting because they suggest that our genetic expression and our physiology are dynamic and highly influenced by our experiences and our sense of control over them, respectively. You can decide whether you live in health and wellness or you cause our own demise by how you think, act, and eat, or your capacity to love or show empathy, etc.

The literature in psychoneuroimmunology continues to support that what you think or feel can have effects on your nervous and endocrine systems and thus, your whole body and your health, especially over long-term periods.

If you think in a negative or pessimistic way, your gene expression should be reflective of this psychological state, just like if you think in a positive or optimistic way. Studies show that your gene expression changes with your mental or emotional state and with your psychosocial interactions.[102,103,104,105,106,107]

Even your immune system shows decrements in performance and cell counts due to a greater pessimistic attitude.[108] Indeed, stress and feelings of helplessness in humans can have similar effects. Thoughts, emotions, and life experiences can have an effect on immune function, neurochemistry, endocrine function, anatomy of neurons, and mental illness, etc.

In other words, how you live matters. What habits you cultivate matter. When your levels of stress are too high, especially when perceived as uncontrollable, any adversity, or persistent thought or emotional pattern can have a profound effect on your health and overall well-being by adapting your body to either positive or negative states. This can happen through a variety of systems, including the immune system.

The SNS appears to be one of the keys that unlocks the doors toward immunosuppression, inflammation, or disease. Therefore, you must find a way to decrease its activity and of other stressful or inflammatory pathways to bring balance, energy, and power back into your being.

Final Thoughts

You are the architect of your body. You can choose how your body develops, adapts, and changes over time. Life changes often require adaptation and thus can be stressful and cause suffering. Even moderate or trivial obstacles can become bigger problems if not handled with perspective and balance. Change is an integral part of life, not a threat to your being, and you must remain adaptable and flexible for success in managing stress levels.

All too often, it is an unbalanced view of a situation that leads to maladaptive responses. You can respond in a more adaptable way by learning to bring to your day-to-day activities the mindful awareness that you can learn by cultivating some of the practices described later in the book.

Take a pause to regroup and observe those stressful moments with care and detachment. These should not cause you to lose yourself. Maintain your center of balance to retain tranquility of body, mind, and spirit. Do not let the situation in the exterior have so much power over you and cause you to lose yourself through the senses and out on to the world.

You can learn to collect your energies and harness them to avoid this diffusing process. See these stressful situations more as challenges that are testing your resilience and resolve. Ground yourself in your body and breath moment-to-moment. As you become aware of your body through the practices of this program, you will bring that awareness during the moments that push your buttons.

Where are you holding tension? Are you checking into how your breathing is doing? Has your heart rate picked up? What emotions are being stirred up inside? By bringing these types of thoughts into conscious awareness, you can then channel the energy stirring inside and about to explode uncontrollably in an appropriate, healthy, and measured way. You can gain dominion over any force once you become aware of its presence and learn how to neutralize it at the source with simple yet effective techniques.

Chapter 6:

Unwinding the Knots

"Breath is the power behind all things...I breathe in
and know that good things will happen."

— Tao Porchon-Lynch

Beginning to Neutralize Stress

I know that you can overcome stress and respond in a different way. You can catch the stress reaction early enough to prevent a circumstance or event from turning into a full-blown stress or anger episode, and instead respond with control. Control, however, without suppressing your emotions, but by learning how to work with all your reactions. You learn to let yourself be controlled less by your emotions by reacting more effectively.

If you do not find ways to relax, you will just keep going and going throughout the day and bypass the processes of rest and rejuvenation, which then reflects in your inability to get good quality sleep at the end of day and in your reactive response patterns. For thousands of years, yoga and Buddhism have offered a number of techniques and practices to influence your autonomic nervous system and elicit a strong relaxation response, improve your attention, increase your awareness, cultivate peace and tranquility, etc.

Inducing a strong relaxation response is key as it relates to stress reduction. Dr. Herbert Benson, one of the fathers of mind-body medicine and a professor at Harvard Medical School, first coined this term. The relaxation response is a state that can be achieved through a variety of yogic practices, including meditation.

As you would expect, the relaxation response reduces SNS responsivity by reducing the effects of norepinephrine.[109,110] In addition, the relaxation response, can, like stress, elicit gene expression changes, but ones that are beneficial to our health and well-being. For example, it changes energy metabolism, enhances the functions of a crucial organelle in cells called the mitochondria, improves insulin secretion, helps to maintain the ends of chromosomes intact (which is thought to be involved in aging – less telomere fraying), and decreases inflammatory and stress-related pathways.[111]

People who take charge and begin a mind-body program for learning to reduce stress and increase relaxation end up being more resilient, taking ownership of their own health by doing what is better for them starting at home, and using 43% fewer medical services than the year before.[112] Even though participants enrolled in eight-week programs show better results, you can, even with as few as ten to fifteen minutes of practice, show improvement, but consistency is the key. If you get organized and commit to yourself, there is no reason you cannot integrate a healthy program into your daily schedule.

You could begin the day with a relaxing yoga posture sequence (See Appendix A for a morning Yin yoga routine. At midday or at any point you find your stress levels rising, close your eyes, tune into your breath, and work on making it deeper, slower, and with a longer exhale, as you visualize stress leaving as darkness, and relaxation and energy coming in with the inhale as light.

You could also, while at your desk, for example, tune into your body and scan it from the feet up with eyes closed, and again take deep and slow breaths while noticing the bodily sensations (i.e., heart rate, muscle tension) and trying to bring your body into balance. Even a five-minute break a couple of times at work would do wonders, not only for your health, but also your productivity. Finally, why could you not end the day with a mindfulness practice, guided meditation, or a yoga *nidra* routine that works for you, if even for ten to fifteen minutes?

Meditation is something that people often find laborious and tedious, even though it is a proven antidote for many chronic ailments, including for reducing stress and anxiety, elevating the mood, and reducing fear. Meditation may be able to do this by modulating the levels of various neurochemicals, including gamma-aminobutyric acid (GABA), melatonin, and norepinephrine to reduce anxiety; serotonin to elevate the mood and counter depression often seen with chronic stress; or modulated dopamine levels to help diminish fear, lack of motivation, and restlessness.[113] Mindfulness meditation in particular as a form of attention training has been shown to help lower anxiety by helping subjects more easily shift their attention away from threatening stimuli that could induce a stress response.[114]

Remember that the relaxation response depends, at least in part, on the activation of the PNS and a turning down of the overactive SNS, thus bringing the person into balance. The practices mentioned throughout the chapters and Appendix A serve to do just this, but must be practiced skillfully, mindfully, and with control and care. Therefore, it is often advisable for a beginner to get help from an experienced person who can help him or her integrate these practices at home and at work, and to learn a full routine in addition to therapeutic or Yin yoga postures.

As you increase your consistency in these practices, you disengage from the fight-or-flight response and engage rest and rejuvenation processes. Whether it is therapeutic, mindful, or Yin yoga *asana* practice, getting regular massages, practicing tai chi, or other practices described later on in the book, you must find time to de-stress and recover to avoid long-term built up effects. Consistency in your practices induces a systemic condition that goes beyond just PNS activation and gets a person into a physiological state of self-induced, deep relaxation that carries over throughout the day and makes further improvements ever more possible.

Body Scanning

Body scan meditation is a practice of moment-to-moment awareness of body and anything that you may feel or sense as you sit or lie still and concentrate. I recommend integrating a body scan practice into the eight-week program early on to help deal with stress, anxiety, tension, or physical pain.

Ideally, during a body scan you scan each body part with eyes closed, starting with the left foot and culminating with the head and scalp region.[115] As you move through scanning the body, you will discover feelings or sensations that you may not like, such as pain, irritation, discomfort, sadness, boredom, numbness, etc. Instead of escaping or distracting yourself from an unpleasantness or even wrestling with it, you learn to gently work through these moments of discomfort or pain.

In the process, you become more appreciative of yourself, accepting of your moments of dysfunction or disability, tolerant of pain (including in others), and able to push through difficult moments with patience and greater care. You may even find that your pain lessens as you learn to let go of the mental grip you have around the site of pain and let energy flow more freely past it. You may often get stuck and lose sight of the fact that everything in life changes. It is often when you hold onto pleasant moments and do not want them to go away, or when you reject painful ones, that you increase your stress levels.

The practice of body scanning will provide you many additional benefits, including: (1) bringing greater awareness to the body and sites of bound energy or tension, (2) noticing a connection between certain emotions and physical sensations, such as pain or discomfort, (3) teaching you that you can work through pain, whether physical or emotional, and (4) training your attention by moving the mind over a body part and holding it there while avoiding distractions.

Body scanning techniques can really be done at any point, whether seated or lying down, whether at home or at work. Initially, however, it should be practiced lying down to develop the mindful awareness required in a calm and quiet setting. Body scanning meditations are designed to help you identify those regions of tension in your body where you have locked up or held excess or inappropriately channeled energies, which is common for someone who is often feeling stressed or anxious.

Typically, you should set aside twenty to forty-five mins for your practice of body scanning, but more is also welcome. This practice can also be done during yoga *nidra*, which I will describe in Chapter 8. If you can, try to fit in at least three separate sessions a week for a month or longer. Research has shown that the longer you practice body scanning, the greater the benefits. With consistent practice, you can help reduce stress, enhance your well-being, and decrease any ache or pain caused by neuromuscular tension.

If you are new to body scanning meditation, then you may want to use an audio recording to guide you until you can do it by yourself. These are available on the internet from a variety of sources. If you find that you are having a difficult time staying awake, consider doing it while in a seated posture.

Begin by closing your eyes to allow you to focus on bodily sensations. Bring awareness to the breath as it moves in and out. However, unlike other practices I will describe, attention should shift to different parts of the body. I often do this for students during relaxation pose (*savasana*) at the end of a yoga *asana* class to help bring awareness to regions of tension where they are mentally or emotionally gripping the body. Allow as much time as you want or need as you experience and observe internally each body area. Some areas may require more attention to fully release the tension stored in them. It is often advisable to have a person (not a recording) guide you through the body scan, especially someone with sufficient knowhow and power of will to induce deeper relaxation states in the person, similar to hypnosis, allowing for greater healing to occur.

After spending a few minutes to center yourself with your breath, move your attention to whichever body area you want. I recommend that you start at your left hand and move up to the shoulder a section at a time (i.e., hand, wrist, forearm, upper arm, and shoulder), then the right hand and do the same as you reach the right shoulder. From there, move to the left foot all the way to your left hip and buttocks (i.e., left foot, ankle, calf, upper leg, hip, and buttocks), and then switch to the right leg and do the same. Your arms and legs should now be fully relaxed and should remain motionless throughout.

Now move to your upper body, back, and shoulder blade region as you move down to the middle and lower back. Swing to your ventral side and take time to observe the abdomen as you move your attention upwards. From the abdomen, move to the chest, neck, face, and scalp. At the face, and even hands and feet, focus on specific micro areas. For example, individual digits in hands and feet along with the top and bottom of your feet and hands. For the face, move through each part of the face one at a time starting at the chin. Keep using affirmations throughout and your power of concentration to bring stress relief and reduced tension.

You can use affirmations to suggest your muscles remain motionless, relaxed, loose, sinking down, and dead-like. In addition, you must remain vigilant to not let your mind wander and lose sight of the body part you are working on. Keep training the mind and it will wander less, giving you greater power of concentration and will. Be like a shepherd gently coaxing the mind, like the herd, back in line. Remember that a mind that wanders constantly is an unhappy mind, and one that is missing the great moments right in front of us in the here and now.

At the end of your body scanning practice, take a few minutes before opening your eyes and sitting up (if lying down), and try to expand your awareness of the entire body as you breathe freely and calmly. Stretch your body to activate your limbs like you would in the morning when you wake up and open your eyes. Try to remain just as present and mindful as you were during this practice throughout the rest of the day.

Body scans or a related version called yoga *nidra* (Chapter 8) are excellent to do in the afternoon when you need recharging and de-stressing to give your family a better version of you. However, remember that for best results, you must avoid falling asleep. Otherwise, you are just taking a catnap!

Positive affirmations at the start of the practice or sitting rather than lying down can help in this regard. Practicing body scanning or yoga *nidra* regularly can enhance your ability to be more attentive to moments in the present and how they may be impacting your body. Additionally, yoga *nidra* can be a prelude to more advanced meditation techniques (higher forms of meditation not discussed in this book).

Working with the Breath

Your breath can be your ally to help bring you back to the present, stabilize and calm your mind, and reduce agitation and overactivation of the SNS (*rajas*). Your breath reflects your inner world. If you feel anxious or stressed, your breath will be broken, uneven, and choppy. On the other hand, when feeling relaxed and focused, your breath will be more even, smooth, and deep, similar to when you are sleeping peacefully. Breathing in a dysfunctional way is often a consequence of stress. The type of inefficient breathing seen during stress can cause tension and uneasiness.

Observing your breath at any given moment can tune you into the current state of your body and mind. Breath control can be a very valuable tool during times of stress. For example, you can tune into the breath during the middle of work or a deadline to bring relief from stress. In this case, you can slow down your breath and make it more regular and extend the exhale to reduce the feelings of stress, anxiety, or panic. While you breathe, try to remain very calm and focused on your breath, and consider using some of the positive affirmations or mantras discussed in this book, or learn from a competent teacher or master.

Breath awareness will immediately draw your focus inwards and away from the source of the stimuli triggering the stress response and toward a state of rest and relaxation. Your breath is often a focal point of concentration during certain meditation practices, including mindfulness techniques. Since the breath is with you at every moment, tuning into it can immediately bring you into the present, where you will be less likely to focus on past problems or future deadlines looming. If you work on bringing yourself back into the present, a new world emerges that you have been missing because of the noise and distraction coming from your thoughts and preoccupations.

Right vs. Left Nostril: Does it matter?

Previously, I mentioned the predictable oscillation that occurs in our nasal passageways. Our nostrils alternatively swell and open, changing from one nostril to the other during the course of the day. In 1895, German doctor Richard Kayser first described the oscillatory nature of our breath. He observed how there existed a nasal cycle of alternating congestion and decongestion that switched between each nostril. In other words, when the right nostril is decongested and open, like during the peak morning hours of alertness, activity, and energy (*rajas*), the left nostril is congested. Conversely, when it is close to nighttime the left nostril should be decongested and open more, while the right nostril should be more congested and swollen in sinuses to promote relaxation and sleepiness (*tamas*). Thus, at any given moment, when you are breathing, one nostril is dominant, and, later on, it switches. As it switches, which does not happen instantly, both nostrils may seem to be in balance and equally active and open.

This alternation makes sense if you consider the nervous innervation coming from the SNS and PNS. The nose region receives innervation from these nervous systems, one covering the right side and another the left. These fibers have opposing effects (sympathetic vs. parasympathetic dominance).

Since the activity of the SNS and PNS has strong effects on your mind and body, control of your breathing through one nostril or the other can influence your alertness, energy level, arousal, etc. In other words, to emphasize the qualities of one of these systems using the breath, you can preferentially breathe through one nostril to increase its associated functions.[116]

For example, if you are feeling sluggish or lethargic, and have low body temperature in the morning and want to initiate a morning meditation practice, let's say, then you will want to practice a breathing technique (*Surya bhedana kumbhaka;*[117] see description in next section) that emphasizes the right nostril to increase heat, blood pressure, energy mobilization to the brain, etc. By inhaling only through right nostril, you stimulate the solar channel connected to the SNS, and by exhaling out through the left nostril, you sedate the lunar channel connected to the PNS.

Conversely, if it is nighttime or you are feeling stressed and agitated, then accentuating the cooling and calming effects of the left nostril would be beneficial. In this case, you would practice *Chandra bhedana kumbhaka.* By inhaling only through the left nostril, you stimulate the lunar channel, and by exhaling through right nostril, you sedate the solar pathway. The differential effects of uninostril breathing have been supported by research studies showing that air flow through the right nostril, for example, serves an activation role through the SNS, while the left nostril relaxes through the PNS.[118,119]

Nadi sodhana pranayama (see description below), where you alternate breathing through the right and left nostrils, can help balance your mood, concentration, and nervous and endocrine systems, lower blood pressure, reduce heart rate, stimulate alertness and focus, etc. *Nadi sodhana pranayama* is an ideal practice at all times and is a perfect prelude to any meditation practice. This breathing exercise serves to balance the SNS and PNS simultaneously, while increasing the latter system's activity more to induce a calming and focused state that is ideal for seated meditation.[120,121] In addition, holding your breath in between alternations serves to energize the mind and body, making it ideal to counter lethargy or inertia (*tamas*) often experienced late at night or very early in the morning. At such times, you can often struggle with remaining aroused and alert.

Reverse Breathing

When you breathe in a normal, healthy way, the abdomen will move out as you inhale and in as you exhale. The abdomen moves out as the diaphragm relaxes and moves down into the abdominal cavity, drawing air into the lungs, and it moves into the thoracic cavity during exhale as the diaphragm contracts. Sometimes a person can get into a reverse pattern where the diaphragm contracts when it should relax and vice versa. Thus, reverse breathing causes the abdomen to go in during inhale and out during exhale, working against the person.

If you turn out to be doing this, there is no need to worry. This is certainly something that you can change over time. You may not know this, but it is likely that, if you achieve deep relaxation as you do when you sleep, you are actually breathing diaphragmatically. You have it already but are putting obstacles in the way during the day, more than likely due to stress and worry.

If you do notice that you are holding tension in the abdomen and disrupting the movement of the diaphragm, then try lying down, placing your hands on your abdomen, and bringing awareness there. In addition, bring love, care, and acceptance there, especially since our culture tends to view the abdomen negatively if it is not perfectly flat. Remember that regardless of its shape, the navel region contains the solar plexus, which possesses immense power if you learn to tap into it.

Diaphragmatic Breathing

Lie on your back and relax onto the floor. Bring awareness to the abdominal region and let the abdomen soften and relax. Observe the abdomen as you inhale (rise) and as you exhale (descend). Let your body relax more deeply. Try to connect to the diaphragm and feel its contraction and relaxation. Practice for five to ten minutes.

For improving the efficiency of your diaphragm during breathing, place a ten-pound sandbag (or a bag of rice) on your upper abdomen. As you exhale, the bag will help expel the air out quickly. Try to resist that consciously to train and strengthen the diaphragm. As you inhale, you will encounter some resistance, which is also good training. Try to make the inhale and exhale equal in length. This will help bring mindfulness to your diaphragm and better control of abdominal breathing. Once you have done this for five to ten minutes, remove the sandbag and notice any changes. Breathing will be much easier (See Appendix A).

Lastly, you can also try *makrasana* (or crocodile breathing) by lying on your stomach with your legs stretched out and your forehead resting on your arms (See Appendix A). Bring your awareness again to the diaphragm as your breath flows in and out. Take this moment to let go of any worry and enjoy yourself. Try to relax and let go of your to do list. All of that can wait the five to ten minutes you practice this. While you exhale, consciously allow the abdomen to soften onto the floor. While you inhale, try not to resist the expansion of the abdomen. Let your airflow move in and out without pause in between. Practice mindfulness by being present with the breath. If any thought or preoccupation arises, acknowledge it, let it go, and go back to attending to the breath.

Note: Please make sure that you make your breath deep, long, and smooth, whether you are doing the breathing exercises lying down or sitting up. Deep breathing will help relax and energize you. The deeper you breathe, the more oxygen and energy that you deliver to your cells.

Breathing Techniques for Balance

Vishnu mudra: This is a specific yogic method that is used for closing your nostrils during the breathing techniques described in the sections below. Use your right hand to close the opening of your nostrils. You will use the thumb and ring finger to press and close the right and left nostrils, respectively, during breathing techniques. Fold the index and middle fingers over the pad of the thumb. Alternatively, you can keep your index finger unbent with the tip resting in the space in between the eyebrows (see photos of the two different versions in Appendix A). The latter is my preferred method as that is how my guru in the Himalayas taught me many incarnations ago. The latter also helps support the head during the chin lock (see below) and draws attention to the space in between your eyebrows, which is a recommended concentration spot (also known as the spiritual eye). The left hand should be resting on the leg in *jnana mudra* to keep subtle energies circulating back to you and not dissipating out through the fingertips (Appendix A).

Surya bhedana kumbhaka: In this method of breathing, you will only inhale through the right nostril. You will want to inhale through the right nostril to full capacity while controlling the inhale by using a yogic technique of contracting your throat called *ujjayi* breath. You will also want to inhale slowly, taking at least five seconds, if possible.

Once you have completed the inhale, you can swallow, retain your breath (*kumbhaka*), and bring the chin to the chest for a muscle lock called, in yoga, *jalandhara bandha*. This *bandha* helps control the energy or vital force as it moves upward and reduces head pressure.

Retain your breath only as long as comfortable without fatiguing but avoid or reduce retention time if you start to feel more anxious or agitated, you have a headache, or suffer from migraines or hypertension. After retention, release the air carefully with a controlled, unbroken, and continuous exhale using *ujjayi breathing* technique (with slightly closed glottis).

Repeat this sequence again, and practice the technique for at least five minutes, or until you feel your body getting warm with some mild perspiration, and your alertness and brain arousal are at a level akin to the middle of the morning or whenever your energy level and attention are at their peak. At that point, practicing meditation, yoga *asana*, or a mindfulness technique becomes advisable and fruitful, especially early in the morning when sleep has made our body and mind slow, cold, and inert.

Ideally, start your practice with ten *pranayamas* a day and build, if advanced enough, all the way to eighty per day. During retention, it is also advisable to maintain some degree of control and tension in the abdominal muscles. In this way, you regulate your breathing better, and more easily expunge lethargy and inertia.

Chandra bhedhana kumbhaka: Practice this breathing technique in the same way, but, as I mentioned previously, inhale with your left nostril and exhale with your right. Again, be mindful of how you are feeling to determine length of *kumbhaka* or retention. This breathing technique offers great benefits for the anxious type of person, as it is a great stress reducer and relaxer.

Nadi sodhana pranayama: This breathing technique is not only great for balancing the SNS and PNS and activating the PNS slightly more to induce relaxation, but also serves as an excellent purifier of nerves (*nadis*). This technique has greater benefits the longer it is practiced.

If practicing during daylight hours, begin this *pranayama* by closing the right nostril with the right thumb and exhaling completely through the left (the opposite if at night or in the very early morning hours, meaning that you start inhaling through your right nostril). After exhaling, inhale for at least three to six seconds depending on advancement (can be longer as well), then cover your left nostril with your ring finger and hold your breath like in the previous two techniques.

Hold your breath ideally for two to four times the length of inhale while doing *jalandhara bandha*. Then release the thumb and the chin lock, and exhale through the right nostril, controlling the exhale and making it twice as long as the inhale (*ujjayi breath*). Then go in the opposite direction by inhaling through the right nostril, retaining breath, and exhaling through the left to complete one cycle. Alternatively, after exhaling through the right nostril to complete one cycle, you can inhale through the left again by plugging the right nostril with your thumb and releasing the ring finger from the left to begin another cycle.

With the help of a competent teacher, you can integrate *kumbhaka* with the different kinds of muscle locks or *bandhas* and concentration techniques. However, for now, use the technique as described above. Also, work toward perfecting the technique by reaching ideally a ratio of 1:4:2 (inhale:retention:exhale). For example, inhale for three seconds, hold for twelve seconds, and exhale for six seconds. I prefer at least 5:20:10, but the longer you retain breath the more taxing it can be. You want to make sure that you feel comfortable and are not fatiguing, and that you keep your head straight and aligned with your spinal cord unless doing chin lock. Breathe smoothly and silently at all times.

Nadi sodhana is the king of the breathing techniques. Yoga students often learn this technique early on in their practice and carry it in their practice throughout their lifetime. *Nadi sodhana* is great at purifying the subtle channels and nerves, and you can couple it with other *bandhas* in addition to *jalandhara*, breath retention after exhale, concentration techniques, and mantras to provide a person with a truly holistic breathing practice. It is outside the scope of this book to go into more details, but a more advanced student seeking help to perfect this *pranayama* can contact me at any point by visiting ramasrootedtree.com.

Note: Ideally, you should practice these *pranayama* techniques seated on the floor in your favorite seated posture (i.e., *padmasana* or *siddhasana*; see Appendix A, for different seated postures) or on a cushion. If that is not possible, you can sit on a chair. Lying down is not ideal, especially with retention of the breath, as it can build up excessive pressure in the eyes and brain.

I often combine various breathing techniques into one sitting prior to the practice of *dharana* (concentration) or *dhyana* (meditation). However, this can take more time than you may have depending on the day. If you are a beginner, use the techniques as described above for reducing stress, increasing alertness, and improving balance.

Again, remember to breathe and be aware of your breath, visualize peace and light suffusing your entire being. Enjoy the breath more and use it to help release tension, stress, and conflict in your body. Practice mindful breathing before coming into contact with painful emotions that may arise during meditation and introspection to make it easier to release them.

Also, remember that you should listen to your body and observe it during these breathing exercises for signs of tension or energy blocks, especially during breath retention. As you practice more mindfulness in every one of your activities or during your *asana* practice, you will become more attuned with your body and better able to know if you should retain your breath, try a different technique, relax a specific region, etc.

Walking with Mindfulness

This is a practice you can do wherever you are. When at home, find a space to either walk slowly back and forth or go to your backyard or a quiet park nearby. You can even integrate this at work (Chapter 7) or go on a nature trail walk while keeping yourself grounded and mindful of your breath and your movements.

The practice is very simple. When you breathe in, you take one step, and when you breathe out, you take another step. Do it with control of breath and step, going as slowly as possible. Be aware of the movement and how it feels in the joints and the contact between the soles of your feet and the ground. Doing this practice barefoot is better, but certainly not mandatory, especially when potentially not appropriate, like at work. Think with one step: "I am present," and with the next step: "I am here." Think these words with purpose and not just as mere statements.

The awareness of each step represents your statement that you are present in the here and now. That you accept yourself as you are in the here and now. The past and future do not matter in that moment. In fact, they do not exist. Ground yourself with each step, as you dig into the ground and grasp it with your toes and imagine you are forging a new path, a new destiny for yourself. This is the complete antithesis of your everyday life where you rush through life doing and thinking, distracted from the greatest gift you have: The Real You. As you slow down your walking and bring mindfulness to it, you reign in your mind and anchor yourself to the here and now. If thoughts permeate your awareness and want to sweep you away, you avoid going into the past or future, or into fantasy or daydreams by the power of your mindfulness that draws you gently into the present without judgments or longing.

Additionally, you can practice this when walking to work or anywhere else. Instead of walking so slowly, take three to five steps per inhale/exhale and maybe do not breathe as slowly. Nobody has to know that as you walk you are being mindful of your every movement and every breath. This will reinforce the practices you do at home, thus increasing the power of your concentration and will.

Self-Healing or *Abhyanga*

As I mentioned earlier, massage can be a great component to your wellness care regime even if you lack a knowledgeable pair of hands to give you what your body and mind crave. Do not waste time desiring to go get a massage if you cannot afford it or find the time. You can show love and care to yourself right now. With time, your partner can also help with building a connection by giving you a relaxing massage you deserve, and you can do the same for him or her. Massage decreases levels of the stress hormone cortisol and increases the levels of two key neuromodulators, serotonin and dopamine, to help elevate mood and enhance motivation, drive, and pleasure.[122]

Therefore, finding a way to self-heal with your own hands or your own movements can be helpful. Your hands can be powerful sources of healing, vital energy that you can deliver to your own body or to another. Why not put this into practice for your own benefit? Unlike a masseuse who cannot get feedback on ideal pressure, as you work on a region, let us say your feet, you can apply it to the right region and with the right pressure.

Remember again to be mindful by closing your eyes and being aware of your body and areas of tension. By bringing the energy of mindfulness during any practice, you increase relaxation and bring greater power to your prefrontal cortex for increased attention and inner control.

There are a number of gentle poses you can do with movement to massage your back (i.e., rocking, rolling, or twisting; see Appendix A). Not only can you do gentle therapeutic yoga postures, but you can also massage your body directly with your own hands. This type of self-care will enhance your mood and self-esteem, and reduce the impact that stress has on your body and mind.

The ideal time to do self-massage is in the morning before showering, even if it means only fitting in the time to do your feet and/or scalp and neck. However, you can also do this before bed to help with sleeping, especially if you are struggling with anxiety or insomnia. Warm some sesame oil[123] by placing the oil bottle in warm water or, if you live in warmer climates, just use it at room temperature.

Place a towel where you are going to sit or stand. Apply small amounts of oil to your hands and massage it onto the area of focus. You can start with your feet and work your way all the way up to your scalp. If applying to the scalp area, applying amla oil is great to use at night for enhancing hair growth and slowing down the signs of aging (greying of hair). If you do use amla oil on your scalp, then leave it overnight and wash it off in the morning.

Always try to massage with upward strokes to counter the effects of gravity, which pulls on your skin on a day-to-day basis. When massaging the abdomen, use clockwise movements to stimulate elimination and counter constipation. Afterwards, shower with gentle soap and shampoo.

Doing a mini massage if you are short on time can also be effective. Never give yourself less because you feel that five to ten minutes is not enough. For any practice, five to ten minutes here or there is better than nothing. Remember, those breaks you take to nurture your being are moments you break the stress cycle and can heal.

Yoga for Higher Practices

Our go, go, go and do, do, do mentality in the West has made us very goal oriented and driven by power, activity, and a sense of accomplishment. However, if you are to master yoga and overcome stress, you need to learn to slow down and engage your frontal lobe more effectively to enhance higher yogic practices (i.e., meditation) and gain relief from the noise and confusion arising from the exterior. To do this, practice yoga posture sequences in a way that helps to reel in your mind and provide greater control and power, thereby facilitating the practice of meditation.

The way we often go about our lives is how we approach our *asana* practice, like an exercise form only with a strong focus on doing and achieving. Doing an intense yoga practice can be counterproductive for someone who is already stressed out and anxious due to the fact that your sympathetic nervous system will be stimulated further. However, there may be times when a more vigorous practice is recommended, especially for someone struggling with low energy, general lethargy, or depression.

Often, you actually need the opposite of what you think you need to bring you into balance. Going for a five-mile run after a long, stressful day is not ideal in any way, especially for someone with a so-called "Type A Personality." Listen to the natural, intuitive wisdom of your body and give it what it needs, which is often the opposite of what your mind craves.

In general, yoga should be practiced more like Tai Chi than aerobics, where the movements are done with precision, pause, and in sync with breath. In addition, as much as you can, poses should be held for longer while keeping your eyes closed and focused on the space in between your eyebrows, on bodily sensations, the steadiness of your breath, or the flow of subtle energy through the body.

If your movements become more controlled, whether it is while eating or walking, or during speech and writing, you engage your prefrontal cortex and associated regions and begin to gain greater power of concentration and regulation of behavior. This power, impulse control, and higher emotional quotient grants us freedom from the sways of life and the effect that moment-to-moment stresses have over us.

I know that you cannot always be slow and measured, but the more you can practice it the better. In Chapters 7 and 12, I will go into how to integrate more of these mindful practices into your daytime hours to achieve better results long-term and make difficult habits into effortless ones.

This book is not the ideal way to teach an entire sequence of yoga that you would get in an hour and a half class at a studio, but in Appendix A, I do include a some restorative and Yin yoga sequences you can do at home. These also achieve the desired effect of stress reduction while at the same time reinforcing a mental and emotional state conducive to meditation.

Both Therapeutic and Yin yoga practices will help you work at being more accepting without the excessive doing or trying to change things, but instead being with yourself exactly the way you are. If you are able to settle into the pose with your eyes closed, then work at maintaining your attention on the present moment and using the pose as a meditation and your breath as an anchor, which is what it is meant to be. Avoid falling asleep in any of these poses so that you do not diminish the efficacy of the pose. This is why doing invigorating breathing exercises before doing these more internalized *asana* practices can be helpful to energize your nervous system, increase your arousal, and improve your attention.

There are differences between a restorative, therapeutic practice and Yin yoga. Firstly, in a Yin yoga practice, there is a greater load and stretch of your connective tissues that may be a challenge initially to anyone who is lacking flexibility or does not practice yoga often. In Yin yoga, the joint targeted will not be supported, allowing for a deeper stretch. Therapeutic yoga, on the other hand, wants to invite you to relax and feel supported by props that can make healing more accessible.

This does not mean, however, that you cannot achieve deep relaxation and concentration during Yin yoga, but that you have to build tolerance and flexibility first. I myself practice Yin yoga more when I am feeling like I need the restorative aspects of therapeutic yoga, but with a more regular *asana* class feel to it, where I still get some challenging poses in and keep my joints loose and stretched. Either of them is an excellent option, but keep in mind that you have to listen to your body and mind and find what would be of most benefit to you.

In addition, when you practice any yoga *asana* routine, the goal is to move slowly and with longer hold periods in between transitions. Transitions should be done smoothly and with control to avoid interrupting your concentration on whatever you are focused on at that moment, whether it is your breath, the space in between your eyebrows, areas of tension, etcetera. Avoid letting intrusive thoughts or preoccupations distract you and take you away from the here and now. Unless unable to do so, consider closing your eyes to enhance your inner awareness and help bring greater tranquility, especially when coupled with slow, deep breathing, which I mentioned is important to tuning your nervous system and PFC function (Chapter 4).

Of course, working with an experienced teacher will certainly go a long way toward finding out what benefits you the most. General yoga classes are not designed with you in mind because they cannot take into consideration your past, needs, constitution, energy quality, and your own journey of healing and self-discovery. If you are interested in a more personalized yoga practice that would benefit you more and is focused on your own developments and trajectory, find me on social media or visit ramasroot-edtree.com.

Guided Meditation

This meditation is good to do after taming your excessive energies and pervasive thoughts with the breathing techniques previously described. You can also precede this meditation with a yoga *asana* routine or thera-peutic or Yin yoga sequences, like the ones shown in Appendix A. As you feel yourself calming down near the end of your posture practice, transition to *savasana,* or relaxation pose. You can use an eye pillow to reduce stimu-lation and even use soft foam earplugs to drown out any noise.

Avoid falling asleep and, after five minutes of doing a body scan start-ing at the feet and going through your entire body to relax it, transition to sitting directly on the floor, on a cushion, or on a chair with your feet flat on the ground. This is your time to journey inside with loving care and patience. Be fearless and relax. Also, accept that your mind will be an obstacle to reaching peace and quiescence due to a lifetime of mindlessness that many of us cultivate.

Take a few deep breaths and keep your attention fixed on the sensations on your nose. With each inhalation visualize light coming in through your nostrils and down to your lungs. As the breath fills the lungs, visualize that both light up and the light is absorbed into your circulation spreading throughout your body. With each exhale, visualize darkness leaving and with it, all the worry, tension, and heaviness of the day. Inhale light and exhale darkness.

Let the breath be what it may as it flows easily and gently. If you get distracted by thoughts or worries, do not judge the thoughts or let them compel you to stop. Persist through these momentary obstacles, which are normal, especially for a beginner, and bring your attention back to the breath. If thoughts become persistent and intrusive, then add in a mantra. With each inhale think So (sooooooo) and with each exhale, Ham (sounds like huuuuumm). Inhale, sooooooo, and exhale, huuuuumm. To deepen your practice over time, you can move your attention to the space in between your eyebrows, or your spiritual eye. Try to keep focus there for at least five minutes.

With time and continued practice, you can drop the mantra, increase the formal sitting meditation, and maintain an internal focus that slowly withdraws from the exterior and goes deeper within. The goal is to eventually reach a realm of being where you are completely present and free of conditioning, objectivization, or even of putting up substitutions in your mind that only get in the way of feeling at peace and overflowing with bliss.

Persevere in your meditation practice or reach out to someone, like myself, that can help you master this important practice, if you find yourself struggling. Remember that research has shown that meditation is the key to transformation and growth.[124,125] If you do not take the time to just be and explore aspects of yourself that remain veiled, then you are limiting your potential for growth and Self-Realization.

The Story of Chris

Chris was about thirty-five years old when he reached out to me. He was suffering from chronic back and neck pain, which related to years of carrying most of the financial burden in his household and holding improper postures while seated. However, he was not aware of this at the time I spoke to him.

Chris was an active man who regularly exercised and ate well enough. However, his pain would not go away. This was causing him constant frustration and discomfort to the point of limiting him in his normal everyday activities. He was having problems teaching his students and standing for long periods. In addition, he was limited in how he could play with his kids and the exercises he could do when he worked out.

As I started talking to Chris, I learned that he was the kind of person who did not complain much about things and that he did not share his feelings easily with others. If something bothered him, he would rather resolve the issue on his own or keep it bottled up than share it with others so that they could potentially help fix his problem much easier.

I determined that he kept many of his emotions to himself for two main reasons. Firstly, he did not want to be a burden to others around him, including his wife, who was always struggling with anxiety and stress due to work, children, and many other duties. Secondly, he did not want anyone to be upset or disappointed in him when he made a mistake or was in need of help.

One thing that he was missing was a conscious connection to his body. Like many of us, he would go about his day busily, unaware of his posture, how stress would imprint on his body, and how he had built pent up negative energies in specific areas of his neuromusculature. His mental tension could be seen throughout his upper back and neck, where he held a grip on certain muscles. Consequently, these activated nerves caused pain and discomfort. He did not know how to let go of this mental grip nor how to open up to those close to him.

I knew that there was more to this pain than just this. I soon found out that the origin of this grip and closure traced back to his childhood, where he grew up trying to be the perfect child to avoid the wrath and breakdowns of his mother. In addition, he never took time to process daily experiences that accumulated within him as bound energy or tension. He often felt like he did more than the average person did and carried a heavy weight on his back. Without the energy of mindfulness, he lacked the requisite skill to extirpate these mental grips. Moreover, he did not know how to relax, unwind, and release his angst and inner turmoil.

One of the first things I suggested to Chris when he signed up to work with me, was that he needed to see a chiropractor and begin a yoga practice designed by me specifically for him to bring awareness back to his body and breath. I told him that this would help keep him healthy and pain free long-term, but that he needed to make some changes as well.

Over the course of the next eight weeks, I taught Chris a program based on this book, but specifically designed for him, his needs, his constitution, and his body type. I reinforced the idea that he did not need to reach out to the exterior first for his healing, whether it was medication, a massage, or a relaxing trip. None of these were bringing significant relief. He could do this himself with the right lifestyle and self-care tactics, and by bringing mindfulness to his every action.

He struggled at first to embrace this philosophy, having come from a culture used to the quick fix. I stressed to him that he needed to remain patient, push through, and persevere. I knew he would see results if only he persisted with the exercises and practices. He did integrate most of the dietary changes I prescribed but struggled with meditation and other seated practices because he was very stiff and lacked the requisite suppleness to sit for extended periods. He actually took better to body scanning and yoga *nidra*. Therefore, I prepared two recordings specifically for him to work through the areas of tension and loosen the mental grip he had over those regions.

With guided relaxations and further explanations, he realized how he was contributing to the grip. As he drove or worked at his desk, he was able to be more aware of this body and sites of tension. He struggled with mindfulness practices at the start, but with time, he became better versed in bringing his full presence and attention during everyday activities. He improved his posture, learned to use his breath and a mantra to relax, and decreased his reactivity during stressful situations. Moreover, he learned to avoid closing up emotionally as often as he used to when confronted by challenges or difficult people, especially those involving angry emotions that in the past had triggered the expression of a traumatized child.

With time, his relationship with his wife improved as he felt better, complained less, and shared more. He learned to trust those close to him more and look for their support. His ideas that he had to do things alone and had to carry all the weight by himself dissolved with time.

I am very grateful for the opportunity to serve this gentleman and scholar. He is now pain-free and able to share his emotions and fears more freely with his wife. He was able to overcome the inner child trauma that was keeping him prisoner, and live happier and more stress-free.

Chapter 7:

Working Overtime

*"First you have to do all that you can do, and then you have to
learn non-doing. The doing of the non-doing is the greatest doing,
and the effort of effortlessness is the greatest effort."*

— Osho

Changing My Perspective

Stress-related problems arise very often from the pressures we feel at
work. We certainly do not find companies or firms that will put our
interests over their own. Different people with various expectations
may be pulling at us in many directions and draining us of vital resources.

As stress begins to accumulate mostly due to work, we can end up
going to a doctor with a variety of physical or mental complaints, including
upset stomach, headaches, insomnia, depression, anxiety, etc. What
the doctor often does is prescribe something for the symptoms (effects),
tell you that you are just stressed, and not deal with what underlies the
stress (cause).

Therefore, depending on another person for our health is a risky proposition. We should take our health into our own hands to become free of disease and enjoy a happier life. We cannot let work of any kind be the trigger that gets our life spinning out of control, interfering with our ability to relate to our loved ones, sleep well, find time to exercise, take care of ourselves, etc. We can go on like this for years and even go past the breaking point to impact our health in ways that cannot be fully quantified.

For many, work correlates with stress levels and these levels tend to peak during pressure periods like the end of the month when we try to meet the minimum billable hours, or when a certain number of sales have to be met, or when a big project or case is due. Unfortunately, our home is not always a respite from our exposure to stress, and thus our levels of stress may not begin to drop until very late at night, close to bedtime.

No matter what we do for a living, even if we are a stay at home parent, we do not escape the fact that we work for a living and we can perceive our work as stressful. Often, we tolerate a stressful job because it comes with a big paycheck. In addition, even after we get out of work, we still have many other duties to take care of. We work at home: cooking, cleaning, taking care of children, driving them to their activities, paying bills, etc. Certainly, we do work that exposes us to a number of pressures and stressors coming from a plethora of sources.

In addition, the people at work, like a controlling boss or a competitive co-worker, can be a source of immense difficulties, which may frustrate and anger us, fueling the fires of stress pathways in our body. When we get home from a day at work, we may have to deal with a difficult or sick family member, a struggling marriage, or children to care for.

Therefore, we cannot easily escape that work will often be a source of stress. Then how can we navigate through this minefield of potential stress triggers? There is a way to escape the pressure, the overwhelming sense of worry, doubt, or fear that arises during these moments at work and afterwards.

Feeling that you cannot fulfill a duty, or that you will struggle on an upcoming exam, or will not meet a deadline, does not help. Worrying about the what ifs in the future will not reduce your stress levels nor will longing for a different life or a different moment. What you can work on is changing your perspective in the here and now to feel more content with whatever you do for a living.

We sometimes feel like we are working overtime due to having the wrong perspective about work in and out of the house. For others, work feels stressful because they do not like what they do. We find it hard to reconcile our dreams, wants, or desires with what we spend the bulk of our time doing. We wake up, get ourselves ready for work, get the kids ready for school, eventually get to work, and spend six to ten hours working, hustling, and struggling only to keep doing more of the same for others at home, and often feel underappreciated and taken for granted. Eventually, we end the day in bed watching television or reading a book until we pass out, only to start the process all over again.

On the weekends, a different kind of work surfaces, like running a variety of errands, maybe cleaning the home, preparing for the next week, taking the kids to an activity or two, etc. This causes weekends to feel like work as well and leaves us yearning for the next vacation break.

That type of endless cycle that we call life that carries us from youth to retirement is thought of as the norm.

What we can control is our perspective. We work mainly to make money, but it can also be a way to connect with the world, to do a service to society, to do something meaningful.

If we love our job and love what we do, then work may not be as significant a source of stress. But even then, if we are not careful, we may fall victim to stress by taking the wrong approach.

Is it possible to make your passion into your source of income? Certainly. But if you cannot, then you should begin by recognizing every moment as a learning opportunity. You can embrace even the difficult challenges you may face as integral to your growth and development. Remember that, no matter what you do for a living, every job serves a purpose and has meaning. In addition, you get to provide for yourself and your loved ones. Your job, whatever it is, can become something that you choose to do rather than something that you do out of necessity.

Creating a Mindful Workspace

Integrating your spiritual and mindful practices into your workplace and in your daily activities can be very helpful to establish a routine of nurturance, self-care, and growth. Even when you may be in the midst of doing, you are still taking care of yourself, creating the habit of just being, and practicing mindfulness. You do not have to get away from a stressful job for your work life to improve. By simply bringing the peace and joy you cultivate in your home practice to work, you can shift the balance in your favor as you learn to see work as a vehicle to serve, learn, and grow. Obstacles can become fun challenges and opportunities for growth, and frustrating moments can strengthen your will, patience, and tolerance.

Rather than cultivate the destructive and overwhelming energies of stress, build and maintain the energy of mindfulness to keep it working in your favor. Just as you would practice mindful walking (described in the previous chapter), or mindful eating (in Chapter 4), you can challenge yourself to practice mindful working.

Do not just mindlessly plow through your work day and then suffer the consequences later. Bring the inner resources you are developing at home to bear fruit on your working day. Maintain awareness of your posture. Notice what events are triggering you to hold your breath or increase anxiety or worry. What can you do differently? Where are you holding tension while on the computer?

Active introspection and inner analysis of your reactions is important to document what you are sensitive to and what is draining you. You can become more aware of how you hold tension and where. Practice some breathwork for a few minutes to de-stress in the middle of the day or during breaks. As you create these gaps in your work day to recharge and refocus, you create a reserve of energy that helps propel you along and reduces the negative buildup of stress hormones in your body. In addition, you help balance the habit of doing with the principle of being.

A key to this practice is to develop a mindful workspace, especially if you work in an office setting with a desk. Integrate some of the elements of the space at home that you use for your meditation practices. At home, you should have set aside a room or a space that is only used for meditation and other practices to build a psychic environment conducive to healing and concentration. Whether it is burning of incense, some aromatherapy oils, or some inspirational décor, bring this element to your work as well, if possible (i.e., if you have your own office space).

Even preparing a midmorning or afternoon tea to relax your mind, and sipping it with mindful awareness, can be invigorating. Keep treating yourself with respect, care, and love no matter what. I guarantee that taking breaks of these sorts will make you more productive than before, as you will feel more content and energized. In fact, talk to your business or firm and ask human resources or ownership for a workshop at the company or at a company retreat, as this will be a worthwhile investment for them as well. Productivity is bound to increase when employees are happier, have surplus energy, and are more relaxed and focused.

As you improve in your practice in this or another program, others will take notice and may even follow suit. Take a leadership role as you learn through this process and help someone else who may need this as well. This will give greater meaning to your life as service is the greatest form of worship, and, as a Harvard University study showed, leadership is associated with lower stress levels.[126] Thus, find ways to take on a leadership role at work or outside to lower stress and build confidence and purpose.

By bringing your practice into the workplace, you can more clearly see what is happening at work that is throwing you off. As you get more attuned with your body and mind through body scanning techniques or by developing a consistent meditation practice, you will begin to feel for yourself what it is like to be without any conditions or obstacles in the way of the Real You.

In those moments, you can grow accustomed to yourself and recognize where your weaknesses lie. Taking time to reflect on your day in a quiet place can then open the door to new insights into aspects of yourself that you had not noticed. It is possible that during this time of reflection or introspection, you notice how you are still carrying pain or scars from your childhood that affect you today at home and at work, maybe in the way you relate with or treat your children or employees, respectively.

In Appendix A, I have included a series of exercises you can do to keep your body loose and to build great mindfulness at work. These are more examples of opportunities to build positive energies and a greater love toward yourself. By taking moments to nurture yourself, you gain in love, energy, and confidence that will translate into your relationship with others and your productivity at work.

Maintaining Awareness

As you prepare to go to work, do everything at the house with mindfulness engaged, whether it is showering, getting dressed, eating, getting the kids ready, etc. Affirm before you leave the house that this will be a good day at work and that you will work on yourself even while immersed in your duties.

When you say hello or goodbye or have a short conversation with someone, make it count. Do not do it reflexively or hurriedly, without consideration or presence. Show yourself and others the respect that anyone deserves and be fully engaged in the present. Do not continue to alienate yourself in the thought world within. Come out more often instead and engage others with full attention and presence in the here and now.

If you are driving to work or on public transportation, try to take breaks from listening to music, audiobooks, or podcasts. Tune in to your breath during the ride. Walk with greater ease and calmness. Try smiling more and embracing yourself more with love and care as you go about your day to reduce the outer expression of tension and worry. Others will take note of your change and be drawn to you.

At work, continue to monitor your thoughts as often as possible. Notice: where is your mind going, what is distracting it? How are you feeling? Where are your stress levels? If you are keeping a journal (Chapter 12), which I highly recommend at least initially, then write some of your thoughts down to reflect on later.

Develop better habits and integrate them into your breaks. Rather than always getting coffee or spending time in idle talk, try going somewhere quiet to rest the mind and release the inner tension that may have accumulated up to that point.

Interact more with people at work who do not increase your stress levels, maybe someone who makes you laugh or someone who inspires you or enjoys their work. Are the communications at work building stress or bringing you problems? How can you improve your interactions, especially with those who may be rude or hostile toward you? Can you be more welcoming of others and draw them in rather than pushing them away? Is your body language or your voice conveying tension or coldness? This does not apply just at work, as you may even be doing this to your partner at home. Are you taking out your stress and pent up frustrations on him or her?

Make sure to continue to bring awareness to your every movement, whether of your body (i.e., walking, talking, writing, carrying, etc.) or your breath as it moves in and out. Practice your mindful breathing or walking while at work, maybe during a break or before you sit to eat lunch. Make sure to pay attention to those two actions during the course of the day as you effectively train yourself to be present in the here and now. If distracted, again remember to coax your mind back to your breath or steps.

When you breathe in, think: "I have arrived in the present. I am here at the ready." Smile and congratulate yourself with pride and power because being present in the now is a gift. In those moments of presence, you rest and slowly empty your consciousness of turmoil and noise. Try not to think about what you were just doing at work.

Keep training yourself even in these little moments sprinkled throughout the day not to keep running away from your True Self by distracting yourself with the bustle of everyday life. Become a giant and powerful presence in the here and now to amplify the energy and willpower available to you. Just imagine what you could do with that surplus of power at work and at home for yourself and others.

After work, find more time to do things that will de-stress you, like exercise. If the exercise is designed to de-stress you, then even better (Chapter 4). The *asana* practices contained in this book not only bring you balance, energy, strength, concentration, and power, but help to build awareness of your physical body that you likely do not possess right now. Even chiropractic or massage treatments can help in this regard and draw your attention to the sites where you store stressful energy.

As you become more conscious of where and how you hold stress, you can consciously work to let it go and prevent its accumulation in your tissues (i.e., neuromusculature). For example, you may notice how you hold tension, let's say, on your right upper back, shoulder, and neck due to using the mouse on the computer or driving mainly with your right hand. As you notice these fine details, you can consciously adjust your posture, switch hands, roll your shoulders or neck, or even dangle forward in a forward bend (*uttanasana*) to relax the upper body and neck (but not while driving!).

Do Not Let Work Rule You

This could very well be the most important part of this chapter so please pay close attention. Do not sacrifice your lifestyle and happiness anymore. If you are putting work ahead of your well-being, then that needs to stop right now. Your work should not dictate your lifestyle and level of happiness and freedom. There should be no obstacle in the way of prioritizing yourself and your loved ones. There is no paycheck large enough to sacrifice your family, health, happiness, and tranquility. You come first. Do not settle for less.

There are very few businesses that prioritize you. You must do that for yourself without sacrificing your livelihood. Yes, it is possible, but you must start by readjusting your life in a way that fits your needs into your schedule. The more you do this, the happier you will be and the more energy and passion you will possess that can naturally feed into every aspect of your life, including your work.

If life has become work, then make it playful and joyful again like an ageless child. Rediscover the youthful freedom, tranquility, and energy you possessed as a child. I have met many people who had very high stress jobs and left them for jobs that brought them greater joy and fulfillment, while still allowing them to provide for their families. For example, I worked with an attorney who became a high school teacher because her passion was not to be a slave to a firm that did not care about her or her well-being. She instead wanted to inspire young minds toward greatness.

Find your passion and find time for it, even if it is just as a hobby. If your job is not your passion, then make time for your passions and integrate your loved ones in those passions, so that they may see you at your best, radiant and carefree. Help them see and feel your passion and love for life.

Strive toward separating work from home and vice versa. Avoid doing work at home. If that is not possible every day, then limit the work you do, especially when sharing time with your loved ones. They deserve to see you without a laptop or files in the way. Remember that it is not about quantity, but quality.

If you must bring home work on occasion, then do it, and make sure to spend quality time with your loved ones before or after. Do not sacrifice the people who matter and who will be there at the end. Think about who in your life will be there when you are on your deathbed and make sure they are loved, cared for, and given the attention and respect they deserve.

Lastly, avoid bringing your personal problems to work. Avoid ruminating about your marital dispute the night before while preparing a document at work, for example. Focus on work at work and home at home.

These are just suggestions or tips and not necessarily a method per se. Whatever you decide, do what works for you to reduce the stress that is preventing the Real You from shining through.

The Story of Marco

Marco opened up his business several years before I met him, but by the time we started working together, his business was making millions of dollars a year and he had over fifty employees. It seemed to me like Marco was always at a meeting with a potential client, closing a deal, or managing his multimillion-dollar business even when at his home.

Marco was fifty-six years old when he came to me. He had a serious relationship but no children. He was charismatic and funny, an excellent sales person with a sharp mind and wit. He was the type of man that everyone wanted to be with. However, right away as I stared into his eyes, I could tell that, although he was popular and wealthy, he struggled with loneliness and doubt.

Marco liked being in a position of power, as it helped mask his underlying fears and insecurities. He started his business by himself for the most part, a real self-made story! Although this made him proud, it brought a lot of problems and stressors with it.

Marco did not know how to turn over responsibility to others. He readily admitted that he was a "control freak," as he would often say. He felt that if something in the office was done without his direct supervision, somehow it would get messed up, and this would reflect badly upon him. His business was his baby and he was not ready to let go or to let it get a bad reputation. However, this was really causing him a lot of anxiety. He was endlessly doing and putting in long work hours. This was taking a heavy toll on his body and mind to the point where he rarely felt happy and satisfied. It was not unusual for him to work ninety hours or more every week.

The more the business grew the more he worked. He was making a lot of money, but he was not enjoying any of it. His anxiety level was through the roof, he would worry about everything from the biggest things, such as trying to get investors or closing deals, to the smallest things, like whether the mail was opened that day. He was working himself to death and not dedicating enough time for himself.

Due to this, Marco was very moody all the time, and he would take it out on his employees, who were really just trying to do their best. His anxiety was causing him to have constant migraines and panic attacks. At times he found himself resenting the very company that he built from nothing for all of this. He was simply miserable. He had built a very nice business that was now killing him!

Marco was stressed because he could not enjoy his life even though he was very successful and wealthy. When he did go on a vacation, he struggled to let go of the cellphone and laptop. He could be seen on a lounge chair, typing away, instead of letting go and enjoying just being.

He signed up to work with me for the year because he wanted more than just personal transformation. He wanted his business to embody the same culture and mentality that he wanted for himself. He knew that happy and peaceful employees would thrive better and be more productive. He felt he owed his employees at least that much.

Therefore, over the course of the first few months, Marco took to the program I developed for him with zeal and fierce determination. In a way, he was the ideal student because he applied himself to the principles and lessons offered to him the only way he knew how to, the same way that had brought him so many successes in his business.

I taught Marco how to bring the practices on the mat at home to his workplace and taught his employees how to do the same in a number of workshops. I explained to Marco how to build a more Zen-like atmosphere conducive to a higher vibration and greater emotional appeal. The employees took to the changes quite readily, and Marco learned how to manage and delegate more effectively with the controlled energy of mindfulness rather than the sometimes chaotic and anxious energy he had carried with him in the past.

As he grew in the program I had developed for him, Marco learned the value of just being. He could see how failure or struggles in business often start with stress as it zaps energy, focus, and clarity, which are integral to success. He also felt firsthand how stress can even exacerbate his inner fears, diminish his motivation, and keep him boxed into a "comfortable zone" that does not promote greater prosperity and long-term growth.

For Marco, it was even affecting how his employees perceived him and his relationship with work colleagues and his own family members. Taking the time to empty the mind gave him clarity and freedom in the present. He could see more clearly and enhance his creativity and that of his employees. Furthermore, it enhanced his mood and overall energy level, which improved his productivity, vision, and interactions with others.

"Oftentimes," he told me once, "I would seek outside of myself for answers, like searching the internet, strategizing with someone, or reading a book. However, I soon realized that, as I became more in tune with my inner self and increasingly more focused and mindful, I could work out a solution without expending almost any energy, sitting there quietly and still. Creative solutions seem to flow more easily then."

"Nowadays, we never start a meeting without first taking five to ten minutes to just be present in silence, relaxing our minds in the process as we breathe calmly and center ourselves in the moment with the intention of being more engaged, attentive, and creative."

"I never knew that I could discover a more spiritual and peaceful side within myself without the need to sacrifice my power and presence at work. In fact, by being more efficient with my energies, I leave more in reserve to be more creative and thoughtful at work and be more loving and kinder at home. I also find that I can enjoy my time away from work more and sleep better, which has helped to decrease my overall stress levels tenfold."

Chapter 8:

Routines for Relaxation and Sleep

"We will be more successful in all our endeavors if we can let go of the habit of running all the time and take little pauses to relax and re-center ourselves. And we'll also have a lot more joy in living."

— Thich Nhat Hanh

Vicious Cycle

Even though we recognize that we are stressed, we may feel that we can still sleep. However, insomnia is not just about an inability to fall asleep, but also to be unable to stay asleep long enough to feel well rested. If you feel tired during the day and often have trouble falling asleep or fall asleep yet wake up in the middle of the night and then have difficulty falling back asleep, then you may be suffering from sleep maintenance insomnia. At the very least, you may be lacking from sleep quality rather than quantity. Even though stress may not be the only reason you are lacking in sleep, as other conditions could be at play such as depression or chronic pain, it is likely one of the main causes.

Chronic stress decreases one's amount of sleep by inducing a state of hyperarousal where your nervous system is too stimulated, thereby upsetting the balance between sleep and wakefulness, or, as we learned in Chapters 3 and 5, between the PNS and SNS, respectively. Your SNS is likely overactive due to stress and it prevents you from relaxing your mind and being able to let go and fall asleep. Even when you do fall asleep, when you wake up, your mind starts racing again, especially if stress is high and you have extra items on your to-do list.

In general, people suffer from quality of sleep issues more than quantity. You may still end up sleeping six hours or so, but finding that it is broken or shallow and not the kind of rest that is rejuvenating and healing. Chronic stress contributes to glucocorticoid (cortisol) increases, which in turn decreases slow wave sleep, the type of sleep that is the most restorative. Sleep is crucial to reduce the levels of glucocorticoids, which can make it harder for you to fall asleep. Lots of stress triggers a sort of positive feedback loop where it increases glucocorticoids, which in turn decreases sleep, increasing cortisol levels further. Therefore, both the quantity and quality of sleep can be impaired by stress.

The key player in this dysregulation of your sleep cycle is likely the HPA axis,[127,128,129] which as mentioned in Chapter 3, regulates cortisol levels. An overactive HPA axis, as can happen during chronic intermittent stress, is at the heart of this pattern of fragmented sleep cycles, a decrease in slow-wave sleep, and shorter sleep times. Moreover, the HPA-axis is inhibited during slow-wave sleep, which further reinforces the positive feedback loop of stress from less quality sleep to more stress.[130,131,132] In other words, stress increases HPA-axis activity and cortisol levels, which decreases slow-wave sleep that would normally help shut this system down.[133]

You can begin to see how sleep disturbances become a problem and exacerbate other stress-related disorders, such as depression or anxiety, when one is already running on fumes. Furthermore, a lack of sleep can elevate cortisol levels chronically, which further complicates sleeping as levels of this stress hormone tend to increase in the evening or during the early parts of your sleep cycle.[134,135] Therefore, reducing stress and getting better quality sleep becomes crucial to avoid these stress-related changes in cortisol levels, altered neuromodulators like norepinephrine and dopamine, and dysfunction of the HPA axis, all of which can disturb sleep patterns and contribute to mental health issues.

Habits and Diet

A sign of elevated stress is not being able to turn off your mind when trying to fall asleep. Being able to fall asleep is a letting go phenomenon. As much as you would like to, you cannot force yourself to fall asleep. Instead, you just have to create the optimal conditions, so that you may be able to fall asleep. By letting go, you relax and can remain tranquil. However, if you spend the majority of your day not practicing this letting go process by keeping your mind obfuscated and agitated, then when it comes to sleeping you will have a hard time doing so.

By practicing mindfulness and other relaxation and concentration techniques, you can rehearse and master this letting go process, which came so naturally when you were younger and more stress-free. Therefore, during the day, we must challenge ourselves to find the time to practice letting go and just being, to achieve greater calmness and relaxation no matter what the circumstance.

Just think about when you were a young child, how deep and restful your sleep was. Your body nowadays is telling you something about the way you are conducting yourself throughout the day and how you have been ignoring it. As the years went on, your exposure to stress slowly changed your body and mind to the point where your sleep quality diminished and/ or stress responsivity increased. In fact, research shows that insufficient sleep, by acting on stress systems, seems to sensitize us to stress-related disorders.[136] In addition, as you would expect, high workload and stress increases tiredness and impairs sleep possibly through altered patterns of cortisol secretion.[137]

Therefore, as we emphasized in Chapter 6, you must find a balance at work to reduce the allostatic overload, which is the wear and tear on your body and brain that are a direct result of your perception of being "stressed out" and having elevated cortisol levels. Create the right framework in your life to improve the balance and efficiency of your adaptive responses to stress while at the same time minimizing the overactivity of these systems.[138] Sleep duration, not surprisingly, is associated with allostatic load and a number of chronic diseases.[139]

So, what can you do to help yourself? Firstly, establish a regular routine. Go to bed and wake up at the same time every day, or as much as possible. Eat warm, nutritious meals at regular times, as overeating, unhealthy eating, and late-night eating all cause your body to work overtime during the night to detoxify and digest these foods. Avoid taking naps during the day as this will make it harder to fall asleep later.

Create a ritual of relaxation that prepares your nervous system for bed by bringing you into balance, along with your SNS and PNS. Take a warm bath or shower in the evening to make it easier to fall asleep. As much as possible, avoid working within the hour or two before you go to bed or doing something overly stimulating like watching television, especially something filled with violence, turmoil, or fear as these all stimulate you stress response systems. Instead, spend that last hour reading an inspiring book or listening to some relaxing music. Maybe take time to bond with your partner through intimate and soothing conversations or massage with warm oil. All of these will help relax you and prepare you for a better night of sleep.

If you like to sleep on your side, it is advisable to lie on your right side while trying to fall asleep. Remember what I explained in Chapter 6 about left vs. right side dominance as it relates to the left and right nostril and the PNS and SNS, respectively. When you lie on your side, the nostril on top becomes the dominant one while the other slowly closes and becomes congested. If you lie on your right side, the left nostril is higher and will dominate your breathing, inducing PNS stimulation and further relaxation to aid in falling asleep. If you are sick or congested, try using a neti pot before bed to clean sinuses and nostrils, allowing you to breathe better (see Appendix A for illustration).[140]

If you wake up in the middle of the night, avoid standing up, as it activates your SNS, releasing norepinephrine into your bloodstream, stimulating brain activity, and making it harder to fall asleep again. Instead, try some of the techniques described below either sitting or lying down. Alternatively, you can do supported forward bends (see Appendix A).

Sleep-inducing Techniques

Some techniques we described before can help improve sleep quality. The practice of body scanning enhances our ability to deepen our relaxation. When we practice it during non-sleep time hours, we do it typically lying down with the eyes closed and are able to observe where we are gripping the body, which ultimately prevents us from fully relaxing. Regular practice of body scanning and even meditation will naturally enhance our physical and psychological resources to more readily establish an optimal condition of relaxation.[141] In addition, as we get more versed in the practices described throughout this book, we better deal with worry or anxiety, which can often strike at night when we feel restless and cannot help but think about the consequences of losing sleep on the following day.

Inversions: You would be surprised, but reclining or inverted poses like *sarvangasana* or headstand, *pincha mayurasana* or forearm stand, *salamba sarvangasana* or shoulder stand, *adho muhka svanasana* or downward-facing dog, and even something as simple as *viparita karani* or legs up the wall can promote sleep (see Appendix A, for some supported inversions). Roger Cole has shown that these yoga poses induce changes in the blood pressure reflex (baroreflex) that induces relaxation and sleepiness.[142] Therefore, practice of inversions coupled with some of the other techniques listed will certainly help.

So Ham: Another practice that proves to be very beneficial is So-Ham meditation (Chapter 6). The worry and anxiety that can often accompany stress keep your mind agitated at night. This agitation will be felt throughout your body and the stillness to fall asleep will not be possible. To help dissolve this issue, try meditating for at least five to ten minutes before going to bed. Sit on the floor by your bed or on the bed with feet flat to the ground and hands resting on your lap in *jnana mudra* (see Appendix A). Bring your attention to the space in between your eyebrows or your "spiritual eye." Follow your breath as you think "sooooo" during inhale and "huuumm" during exhale. Then lie down on your bed face up and continue the same practice of So-Ham meditation until drowsiness ensues and you let go. Avoid breath retention. You should sleep more soundly.

Reducing anxiety: If worry or anxiety are high, whether it is during the day or near bedtime, try the following technique, either sitting or lying down. Inhale through the nose, exhale through the nose. Inhale through puckered lips, exhale through a relaxed mouth. Inhale through the nose, exhale through a relaxed mouth. Inhale through puckered lips, exhale through the nose to complete one full cycle. Continue to repeat this sequence until agitation diminishes and you feel more relaxed and less overcome with fear, worry, or doubts. Make sure to lengthen the exhale to increase effectiveness.

Sleep inducing: Additionally, try this technique while lying down in bed, again if feeling restless and unable to let go. Inhale and exhale normally a few times as you focus on the breath. Make it long, smooth, and steady. Then after a few minutes, inhale and extend the exhale slowly and imagine you are releasing bottled up tension. Follow that with a two-part inhale (inhale, inhale to fill lungs), followed by the same type of exhale. Then one more normal inhale and exhale like before, followed now by a three-part inhale (inhale, inhale, inhale to fill lungs) with extended exhale and mentally letting go. Again, a normal inhale and exhale, followed by a four-part inhale with exhale. Keep doing this alternating breathing pattern as you build all the way to a ten-part inhale followed by a long exhale. However, you should start feeling drowsy and fall asleep prior to that, maybe around the five- to seven-part inhale.

Keeping it simple: Even a basic breathing with inhalation and extended *ujjayi* exhalation can help. You can retain your breath but do not overdo the length to the point where it taxes you, since this will counter the PNS response and activate the SNS to accelerate your heart rate. The same thing goes for extending the exhale. Focus on keeping both your exhale length and breadth retention comfortable and monitor your heartrate and level of fatigue so as to stimulate the PNS and relaxation.

Lastly, you can try *kriya* meditations (*Shabd and Yuni Kriya*, published previously by David Shannahoff-Khalsa, director of The Research Group for Mind-Body Dynamics at the University of California-San Diego).[143] *Kriya* refers to a set of practices, techniques, or exercises to achieve a set outcome. In the case of these two *kriyas*, the outcome is regulation of sleep and deep relaxation. These techniques have been reported in scientific literature as well.[144]

The Power of Yoga *Nidra*

Even though we will describe it here, yoga *nidra* is meant to be practiced similarly to body scanning. We suggest you seek out a competent teacher or guide to help induce a particular state of deep relaxation and heightened awareness, where powerful affirmations and suggestions can be gently introduced into the practitioner's psyche. Yoga *nidra*, or yogic sleep, is a particular state of consciousness that is very similar to that achieved by higher forms of meditation. Through an intricate form of guided relaxation, the person, while lying down in *savasana* or relaxation pose, will become completely relaxed and systematically aware of the inner world that is often ignored for the most part.

I often prefer yoga *nidra* to meditation and so do many of the Himalayan tradition.[145] The advantage of yoga *nidra*, if you remain conscious, is that you can reach very deep states of consciousness without the need to maintain your back and head in alignment or deal with your legs falling asleep or cramping.

The problem for a beginner, however, is the obvious: you can fall asleep much more easily, which is counterproductive. To help with this, like body scanning, it is recommended that you get the help of an experienced teacher or a voice recording that can bring attention to different areas of the body and different images. In this way, your mind can remain occupied and be guided into a deeper state of consciousness conducive to healing and even Self-Realization in the ripe student.

With yoga *nidra*, you can gain the benefits of deep sleep without the dullness in as little as a few minutes to three-quarters of an hour. Yoga *nidra* can really allow you to empty your body and mind of the heaviness of the day and sit in stillness for an extended period of time, affording you the opportunity to enjoy just being without any conditions, thoughts, bodily awareness, or egoic constraints that limit your full expression. In that state, you can Self-Realize and witness directly your True Self, which is *satchitananda,* or truth-consciousness-bliss. Each time you come back to your bodily awareness after this practice, you will feel different: lighter, happier, freer, kinder, and more wholesome and connected to everyone and everything. The little things will not bother you as much and you will provide a joy and peace that others will tangibly feel.

Natural Remedies for Sleep

One of the first things to do to manage your elevated stress and cortisol levels is to ensure you are receiving proper nutrition. This is why I devoted an entire chapter to healing your body through the right foods and healing, holistic herbs. In this section, we will finish the chapter just by highlighting some natural approaches to improve your sleep.

In terms of proper nutrition, please refer to Chapter 4. In addition, consider consuming whole, plant-based food with vitamins B6, B5, and C, which often become depleted with extended hyperactivity of the adrenal gland and excessive production of cortisol.[146]

Warm milk with decaffeinated tea before bed can help bring peaceful sleep. In particular, you can focus on three key herbs: cardamom, nutmeg, and chamomile. Find a tea with these spices and add some warm, nondairy milk to it. Alternatively, you can warm up the milk and add a pinch of nutmeg and/or cardamom.

Reports in Ayurvedic literature suggests that these to spices have a calming effect that can aid sleep. Cardamom is an adaptogenic spice that helps to balance your *doshas*, or energetic makeup. In low doses, nutmeg can have a calming and de-stressing effect. Even the aroma of cardamom or nutmeg (essential oils) can help with insomnia, restlessness, or anxiety. Lastly, chamomile, possessing the antioxidant called apigenin in abundance, induces sleepiness. Apigenin is able to bind to specific receptors in your brain to decrease anxiety and enhance sleep.[147]

Cherries: Eating cherries as a snack or dessert after dinner can help reduce mental stress and fatigue to reduce sleeping problems. Cherries are considered an anti-depressant food that is also tasty and highly nutritious, as it is loaded with antioxidants and anti-inflammatory chemicals. In addition, cherries are one of the few natural sources of melatonin, which helps to improve sleep duration and quality.[148,149]

A delicious nighttime treat is to combine a cup of unsweetened almond milk with a half cup of cold chamomile tea, reported to help with sleeping, in a blender. Additionally, add a cup of fresh or frozen cherries, a banana for an added natural sweetener rich in tryptophan to boost serotonin and mood, a teaspoon of any seed with omega-3 fatty acids, like chia or flax, and a sweetener or vanilla extract to taste, if desired. Whenever blending, it is best to use a vacuum blender to reduce oxidation.

Tomato juice: Tomato juice contains a wide array of phytonutrients essential for health, but related to sleep, the key nutrient is lycopene. Low levels of lycopene in the blood are associated with shorter periods of sleep and difficulty falling asleep, which reduces your chances of getting into the phase of deeper, quality sleep.[150]

Other sources of lycopene are papaya, watermelon, red peppers, and grapefruit. You could also take lycopene in supplement form, though it is better in raw or cooked form. Raw tomatoes preserve the phytonutrients and provide greater healing. However, cooked tomatoes make the lycopene easier to absorb. Combining tomatoes in a dish with cruciferous vegetables like broccoli seems to enhance absorption of lycopene, not to mention the added health benefits. Even tomato juice with a couple of pinches of nutmeg before dinner helps with sleep.[151]

Healing Herbs: Ashwagandha, mentioned in Chapter 4, reduces cortisol, enhances mood, and reduces anxiety, all of which can improve your ability to sleep soundly. The adaptogenic herb *rhodiola rosea* also modulates cortisol. It can even reduce release of catecholamines that mediate the acute stress response and HPA axis activity that is involved in the long-term response to stress. Other safe herbal sleeping aids include valerian root, lemon balm, hops, and passion flower, although conclusive data about their efficacy is lacking. In particular, a natural supplement of melatonin and valerian root can be effective, especially as a nutritional spray.

To stabilize the HPA axis, you can also consider some of these traditional botanicals, including astralagus, holy basil and maca root (both described in Chapter 4), and licorice, amongst a few others. Some nutritional supplements that may also help are phosphatidylserine and L-theanine.

In summary, a whole-system approach to health and wellness is recommended once again to reclaim your youthful, childlike approach to sleeping and restore the balance of your nervous and endocrine systems to decrease cortisol levels and stress.

Story of Nancy

Nancy is a mother, a wife, an only daughter, and an attorney with her own business and approximately a dozen employees. When she came to me, she was forty-one years old. She was drained, tired, and exhausted. She would keep saying to me that all she did was do and do and more do. She took care of her kids, of her employees, her parents, her husband, her duties, and would often not finish until the middle of the evening.

By the time she went to bed, she was exhausted yet had a million thoughts crossing her mind about things that either she had not done or needed to get done the next day. She had due dates for cases that needed to be filed, various emails from clients that she had not responded to, the kids had special events, practices, projects due, her parents needed help with several things, and all the while she needed remain positive and supportive for her husband, who was also busy himself.

Plain and simple, Nancy was tired! However, by the time she got to bed she was so tired that she would fall asleep in the middle of television shows that she would share with her husband or even in the middle of conversations.

However, this sleep would only last for about two hours and then restlessness and tossing and turning would ensue. Her mind would race on and on to no end. She would worry about things she could not control or resolve at that moment. Despite feeling exhausted, unable to rest her mind, she could not find stability and tranquility to get quality sleep at the end of the day.

Often due dates and things that needed to be done would wake her up in the middle of the night after her husband and children were asleep, and she would remain awake for hours. Nancy was a classic example of what goes wrong with persistent exposure to stress. She would often cycle between moments of anxiety and worry to moments of depression and despair. She had a lot to be thankful for but could not slow down and rest in the present to enjoy what she had.

Not surprisingly, the cycle of not resting the day before only provided the catalyst for less rest the next night. On some occasions, her body and mind would give way on days of less doing and she would fall asleep for longer periods. Unfortunately, her rest on those days was still not the restful deep sleep she so desperately wanted. Instead, it was shallow and full of busy dreams.

Poor Nancy touched my heart because, in many ways, she reminded me of wife, who had experienced similar struggles. She was exhausted and fading fast. Nancy was very stressed because she needed to sleep, and she simply could not.

During our initial consultation, I told her: "Nancy, despite the gravity of any situation I may encounter with a client, I always reassure them that there is a solution, and that together, we can work to make things better. Please trust me and know that we can get you to sleep better. I will teach you the secrets to relaxing, not just at night but at any point during the day as well, so that stress hormones stop accumulating and interfering with your sleep cycle."

She trusted my word and immediately agreed to work as my client and student in the art of healing. I wanted to teach Nancy that the approach she was taking in her life was leading her down a path of self-destruction, but that we could correct it and get her on the path toward self-enlightenment instead.

We made significant changes in her diet, habits, and routine that took into consideration her specific psychobiological functioning, her constitution, and her predominant energy qualities. To get her to rest better she needed a complete overhaul, in a sense. She needed to recapture the balance she had lost, and thus we could not focus just on sleeping aids or techniques, but on many of the approaches discussed throughout this book.

As Nancy progressed through the program I had built for her, I began to notice a change in her demeanor and an increased sense of calmness. She began to value time spent on nurturing herself and in cultivating healthier habits for her body, mind, and spirit. Her entire system began to equilibrate as her neuromodulatory networks and endocrine pathways normalized.

She still struggled at work and at home but was able to stop herself from going too far down the path of anxiety and breakdown. She could reel herself in using a variety of techniques I taught her, helping her remain more centered, grounded, and present. With mindfulness energy at her side, she navigated through the day with greater ease, planning her activities better, and making sure that she fit in time for self-care and healthy lifestyle decisions.

Chapter 9:

Finding Time to Love Yourself

"Don't say you don't have enough time. You have exactly the same number of hours per day that were given to Helen Keller, Pasteur, Michaelangelo, Mother Teresa, Leonardo Da Vinci, Thomas Jefferson, and Albert Einstein."

— H. Jackson Brown Jr

Be Present to Increase Your Time

Your experience of stress is often related to worrying about time or the lack thereof. Time has become one of the most common types of stressors we experience today, as we can often feel that we are short on time to get everything done that we need to. You may worry about getting everything done on your to-do list, or struggle with the fear that you will fail at completing an important task.

There could be a deadline looming and you feel like you do not have enough time to finish the work required, or you may be late for an appointment. Alternatively, you may get stressed because you have too much time ahead of you doing something you do not like to do, like your job. This time pressure can grow worse if there is an important deadline coming up and you are behind, or you have many tests in one week and feel unprepared for them.

We think that overcoming time stress can be accomplished by doing more in less time, not noticing all the while that we are building up pressure and activating stress pathways to a large extent, even if we enjoy what we do for a living. This is especially true for women who are great multitaskers. However, the antidote to this time dilemma is to invest more of your time on yourself, in non-doing, to discover the timeless realm where you exist free of any constraint, tension, worry, or condition. To overcome time stress, you must transcend it altogether, if just for a few minutes a day. Remember that the key is not quantity, but quality with consistency.

To discover real peace and break free from worries about time crunches, you must find inner stillness, not in filling your time with doing so much or looking for it outside of yourself, but in non-doing. As you step out of time, whether even for a few minutes, you gain a sense of tranquility, relaxation, and focus that you can bring back with you when you engage time once again. You will find that you can do more in less time when you do take time just to be present in the here and now.

Remind yourself often that time is a product of your own consciousness and your ability to hold memories that give you the experience of the passage of time. In reality, you are timeless and spaceless. You do not have to be in a state of doing all the time and filling up your mind with thoughts, preoccupations, planning, or worry. It is quite healthy to practice non-doing, which trains our minds to embrace passivity, tranquility, and emptiness, all of which are important traits for gaining a clearer picture of who you really are and to begin to enjoy your own innate inner calmness.

You may be wondering how taking time to just be can help, if you already feel so much pressure to do? What you will find is that when you cultivate some of the practices described in this book, you will gain more confidence, control, calmness, concentration, and power to do more in less time. Doing it happily and peacefully will lead to a freeing up of time rather than less time. In addition, through the practice of mindfulness, you will live more in the present and conserve valuable energy that you often waste ruminating about the past, fantasizing or obsessing about the future, or even daydreaming about what does not even exist.

Setting aside time each day, even just ten to fifteen minutes, for formal meditation practice can be invaluable. You are not being selfish for working on yourself. Your partner and loved ones deserve the best version of you. Stop doing so much in the exterior and running away from your True Self. Turn around and look within to find the source of stability and peace within yourself. By focusing more on being instead of doing, and emptying yourself, you learn to experience, accept, and enjoy yourself as you are. And you know what? Who you are is perfect already. You need only to realize it in the eternal now. You will not find it in the dead past or the undetermined future.

If you do not break the habits that hold you back and limit you, how can you possibly expect to gain this type of freedom from time? Being present in the now frees you from the pressures of time, as when you are doing something you enjoy so much that you lose track of time altogether. In that moment, there is no time and even perception of the passage of time will diminish to the point that you even underestimate the time elapsed.

The Plasticity of Time

This perception of skewed time or of altered passage of time is so real that even your body will experience the effects of time differently. In essence, you would age more slowly by doing more things that you enjoy or doing them with happiness and peace to the point where, in your mind, time vanishes. Since the body is a gross manifestation of the mind, the body, in turn, will experience less passage of time as well. Yes, by doing more things that you enjoy so much that you get lost in the eternal now, you will become freed – albeit temporarily – from the constraints of time, and you can age more slowly than normal.

If another person were to be seated by you and be bored doing something he or she does not enjoy, then they would overestimate time and age more. I have studied this in the past and shown, at least in unpublished, preliminary data, that people in the engaged group significantly underestimate time when performing an activity that they enjoy and are highly engrossed in, compared to those doing an activity they do not enjoy.

This illustrates the power we have over the mind and time. Living in the past or the future is not real, and it only exists in our imagination. By getting fixated in the past or future, we miss what is most precious, the eternal now of the present. In addition, we slow down our thought vibrations enough to crystallize our existence and cause us to age more in a shorter period of time.

Time hastens during periods absent of true awareness of the present, and our body and mind will feel it. By working in the present and infusing it with joy and passion, we slow down time to bring it almost to a near halt, making an hour seem like ten minutes. In other words, doing more of what you love and what brings you joy will inevitably bring you more vitality and health, and preserve your youth for longer. The day will go by quicker and yet you will accomplish more.

Concentrate in the Present

Even if you do not think that time has this level of plasticity or effect, you will find that being in the present more will give you more time as you concentrate more energy into that singular moment rather than diluting your existence between the past, present, and future. A person with a concentrated mind can do the work of multiple diluted individuals. Compare a regular household lightbulb with a laser. What a difference, no? The former is diffused and the other concentrated. The latter can damage the retina in your eye and the other cannot.

Similarly, a 95° F room possesses enough heat energy to start a fire, but why does it not? Because the energy is diffused across the room and not concentrated on a single point. Thus, the practice of concentration is important for stress management because it will make you more time efficient, power-ful, and able to be present and free from the constraints of time. Make your-self more concentrated to unlock the immense power dormant within you.

Nothing can touch a person who lives free from the self-imposed pres-sures of time and can find balance and joy in every moment and in every person. You can have that, and, with practice, we can unlock this together. Live in the present more and not on autopilot. Do not let the speed of everyday life consume your energy and will. Slow down, be content in the moment, and practice non-doing to begin to enjoy being and decrease anxiety, stress, and chronic tension.

Do more out of being, rather than trying to fill in as much time as pos-sible with varied tasks. We will find that often we spend our time on things that are not as productive or valuable. Be at peace and in complete aware-ness of the present so that you can effortlessly move the mountains of your life as if they were nothing.

Why Not Be on Vacation?

Be like Gandhi, who despite working up to fifteen hours a day for many years, when asked when he would take a vacation replied, "I am always on vacation." When you focus on non-doing, calmness, and cheerfulness, your entire being becomes quiet and serene, and you become empty or vacant of turmoil and work, and thus are on vacation and in endless bliss.

Try to stop so much doing and learn to take time just being and relaxing in the present moment to help bring the levels of stress hormones and neu-rochemicals to a balanced level and allow your body to soften and release pent up energies. Furthermore, if you learn to practice meditation or mind-fulness techniques, you will literally rewire and retune your nerve cells and neurochemistry. Effectively, you can become the architect of your own well-being by tuning into your body, changing your mental and emotional relationship with it, and thus changing your gene expression and your moment-to-moment secretions of chemicals in the body. Do not try to fill up all your time with doing, thinking, and talking, but instead start taking more time for yourself to nurture calmness and acceptance so that later on, you can do more with greater tranquility, happiness, and poise.

You can learn to relax your mind and body to allow the beauty of your spirit to manifest more. Getting caught up in the moment-to-moment train of thoughts or events and attaching to them through judgments, rejection, or fear can be overcome with acceptance by viewing all events through a different lens and embracing yourself and others with the love that is the very fabric of your being.

Final Suggestions

Be consistent with your practice, as I have emphasized before. Take a portion of your time, however much that can be, to practice just being, especially through meditation. Protect these valuable moments and do not sacrifice them. You are not being selfish. Others deserve to see the Real You, which can only come by taking time to nurture yourself allowing you to show up more in the present.

Preserve your space and time for some silence and withdrawal of the senses, or *pratyahara*.

Live in the present more to reduce anxiety and time urgency. Make every moment your own through the practice of mindfulness. Be aware of everything you do, avoid hastiness of thought, action, or speech.

Remind yourself that the items on your to-do list can wait. They all do not need to get done that instant or that day. Simplify and organize your life to gain more time. There are things that you are doing that you can cut out or diminish. Figure out what they are, with or without help. Remember that by filling up all your time doing, you do not leave much for yourself to do the things you want, to spend valuable time with the people you love and who love you.

Develop good time management skills. In this era of handheld devices with digital calendars and planners, free yourself of having to think about what you need to do and place everything on your device(s) with reminders and alerts.

If you are a morning person, then schedule the most important tasks that require the greatest concentration for this time of day. Prioritize your tasks and schedule them during the times when you are most productive. Leave the less important tasks for times when you have less energy. Remember that the most important tasks are those that help you reach your goals. Therefore, working on these at peak times is a better investment of your energy.

Be assertive, yet polite in declining to help or do other tasks that you just cannot get done due to other more important duties. It is okay to say no.

Chapter 10:

Doing Your Duties Mindfully

"Every time you are tempted to react in the same old way, ask if you want to be a prisoner of the past or a pioneer of the future."

— Deepak Chopra

Sources of Role Stress

One clear effect of stress is this feeling of pressure caused by having to fulfill a variety of roles. The roles we play in life can certainly put a lot of constraints and demands on us. How we perceive our roles and respond to their demands will determine our level of role stress, or stress experienced due to whatever role or job we perform at work or even at home.

We assume many roles based on self-imposed expectations and those originating from others or an institution or corporation. These expectations we set upon ourselves can impose great limitations on our behavior and demeanor, as we think we should act one way or treat someone in a specific manner when under a specific role.

The problem lies in crosstalk, which is when a role becomes so ingrained or habitual that you do not transition out of it when you should no longer be in that role. For example, at work, you spend lots of time being a manager at a firm, holding high expectations, giving out orders, and expecting a fast turnaround of work results. You may often assume a similar role without even realizing it and find yourself, especially during the first hour or two after getting home, treating your children or partner as employees when it comes to getting homework done or helping out around the house.

With an increasing number of women becoming career conscious and holding high stress jobs, yet still having to wear the hat of being a mother, caretaker, and wife, stress can be at an all-time high. Balancing work and family can become an ordeal, as it leads to irregular work hours or working from home, which can put stress on marriage or take time away from spending it with the children.[152]

At work, our role(s) may create conflicts in our relationship with other coworkers, may influence our career development, etc. At home, the same phenomenon can occur. Maybe you are the disciplinarian with the children, or you manage the finances in the house, roles that brings you stress because you may not enjoy doing them. If we do not switch out of work mode when we get home, it can cause conflict with our spouse or partner as well.

Very often, we run into role conflict, which is when our role, maybe as a supervisor at work, brings us stress from having to meet the demands of two or more groups (i.e., your superiors and those you supervise). Maybe a person at work is a friend, but you are also their supervisor and have to hold them accountable. This can put strain on that relationship at times and cause you stress. This type of stress can impact security if it causes psychological withdrawal, leading to reduced job performance.

Another source of stress related to your role at work is role ambiguity, where you lack a clear understanding of your job responsibilities and what is expected of you, especially if you are new to your job. You may even feel you do not have clarity as to how to get something done that you have never done before, whether at school, home, or work. We are always encountering projects or assignments that are new and require that we learn new roles, strategies, techniques, or procedures. This requires greater energy reserves, as we typically have to overcome inertia to gain momentum as we learn to figure things out.

This lack of role clarity and associated worry and self-doubt can lead to enormous amounts of stress, especially in a job that is already high pressured. Of course, this type of role stress can also lead to a lower level of performance, which can lead to a meeting with a supervisor, further increasing stress due to job security issues.

Improving Your Relationship with Any Role

To begin to overcome role stress, your main objective is to work on being present in the roles you play and see the positivity underlying all these roles. We can very easily fall into the trap of viewing the role or roles we are confined in as being the worst possible. We usually take it further by projecting this distaste out and onto the world by stating resoundingly that nobody has the problems we do, that life is so unfair.

However, what we find when we talk to other people in similar situations is that they do feel stressed and do struggle just like us in managing the different roles they must assume. Additionally, we find that they are also dissatisfied with their job at times and may struggle with their roles inside their household or be disappointed by their lack of freedom. Knowing this from others can put things into perspective and help us realize that we are not alone.

No matter what the role is, whether social, professional, familial, or work-related, you will find any role confining and limiting. No matter what role or persona you may assume, it is clear that none of them are the real you. Lost in the shuffle of these different hats we wear is our innate sense of wholeness and completion. By fragmenting ourselves into specific bundles with specific views, strong beliefs, and domains of doing and acting in the world, we have lost sight of who we really are.

Why can you not be how you normally are when engaged in these roles? That is often a challenge, especially when you hold a position of power. You do not want to manage people who do not respect your position because they see you as too nice or friendly. Therefore, it is often inevitable that we have to assume a certain role at work that we may not necessarily enjoy or want for ourselves or for others. The key is not to let it permeate into other roles or relationships, and for these roles not to take the mantle of who we really are.

Again, adaptability and mindfulness are key ingredients. Adaptability to switch roles quickly when needed and also to let go of these roles when no longer appropriate, because crosstalk can increase stress in our relationships as we project our roles into the wrong situations. Mindfulness can help us overcome the negative effects of role stress by helping us see more clearly, be more aware, and avoid misperceptions.

All too often, we blame our roles for our feelings of anxiety, depression, or discontent. However, recognize that it is okay to be a mother, father, lawyer, doctor, executive, teacher, judge, politician, psychologist, etc. The key is to use mindfulness energy to restore the balance and harmony of who you are and avoid getting stuck in certain roles, or not thriving when conditions change and the previous role you held is no longer as important or required. You may not be able to acclimate yourself to a new situation and therefore get stuck in a role that is no longer demanded of you, leading to stress.

Our personality may dictate success in some roles but not in others. Very few people, if any, are perfected Jacks of all trades. We are developed in some areas, while lacking in others. Maybe running a business is a role that suits us, but being a good communicator is not. In addition, we spend so much time at work, especially if work is a sort of addiction that keeps our mind busy and racing onward, that our mind continues to be full of work details preventing us from relating to our partner or children while at home. You may be there physically, but your mind is elsewhere.

Again, bringing mindfulness to play is crucial to learn how to move from one present moment to the next and avoid getting stuck in roles no longer needed at other points in the day. Mindfulness can also help keep you grounded, helping you stay tuned to the people you love and who love you the most. Adaptability is key to avoid remaining stuck in your work role, for example, and able to operate in your other life roles as well without interference from your work role.

I know you often feel alone and isolated in your suffering, but you are not alone. There are people that care about you and can be of help if you let them. Remember what is most important to you. When at home focus on your home, and when at work, focus on work. You may have to assume a variety of roles or personas but ground yourself in your True Self so as to not lose the stability that it can provide. In the midst of lots of change, year in and year out, your body, your personality, and your environment have all changed, but, if you observe very intently, your True Self, the eternal witness, remains ever constant and immutable.

Connect with the Real You to bring yourself back through many a changing landscape and avoid getting stuck in roles we associate with modes of thinking, doing, and judging, and that can then cause conflict with those we love and increase stress in our lives. Bring more awareness to each role you assume, to function more effectively without the dilemma of getting stuck in a particular role and letting it trickle into other situations where that role is no longer suitable.

Part of the problem may be that your view of the situation is being skewed by your own mind that is very attached to this one way of seeing your situation. Break free from that and serve every role to perfection. Life is a divine play! Thus, enjoy your every role as the supreme actor.

Chapter 11:

Unseen Forces

"Difficulty with healing looked upon in the right way...is called
education. When the mind is brought into harmony the body heals."
— Ron W. Rathbun

The Power of our Words, Thoughts, or Actions

The power of our thoughts and words often goes ignored. To overcome the stress originating from within, our thoughts and words can have a sublime effect when saturated with sincerity, conviction, faith, and intuition. You must discover the way to enliven your inner being with spiritual force, with your own soul vibration.[153]

Excessive or idle talkativeness, gossip, or untruths make your mind and words have little to no power and can even cause long-term harm. Practice of *ahimsa* (non-violence) is key here, as is practicing the rest of the *yamas* and *niyamas*, not described in detail in this book.[154]

You should avoid speaking unpleasant words that may be harmful in any way. Instead, seek to become a person who utters sincerity in your words and affirmations with deep understanding, feeling, and willpower. Find the calm, inner voice that we all have and that can guide you more effectively through any difficult moment with detachment, yet not apathy, and tranquility, yet with firm resolve.

Catch yourself before you lose control over your own energy and self to avoid anger, hostility, or excess heat. Calm and cool yourself using your breath as we explained in Chapter 5. Increase your mindful energy reserve to help reel you in and keep you anchored, pleasant, and under control. Practice expressing your feelings in a healthy, calm, and controlled way to let out the pent-up energy or anger you may feel at times in a way that does not harm you or others.

Monkey Mind

Monkey mind refers to having an unsettled or restless mind. The analogy I make is that of a pet monkey that created lots of raucous chaos and distracted a man from being able to concentrate on his craft. Every time the monkey made noise and jumped around, the man would get upset and yell at the monkey to stop. He does not realize that he does not have control over himself in that scenario, but the outside stimuli, the monkey, does in this case. We go about our day in a similar way with a monkey creating all this noise and preventing us from truly reaching our peak. Remember that a concentrated mind is a powerful mind.

Therefore, we should reduce the inner chatter we often experience as we go about our day to bring clarity to what we do in the present and make us more focused. Remember that a concentrated mind is a powerful mind.

This mindless process can include: (1) reading off your to-do list in your head, (2) making judgments of people or situations in the present, (3) recalling past events, whether positive or hurtful, (4) creating dire "what if" scenarios of the future, (5) daydreaming, and (6) listing real or imaginary fears.

How do you tame your unruly mind? Firstly, practice *mouna* or silence (aloud or internal) at least once a week for a few hours to pacify your mind and break the habit of excessive mental verbiage. If you find that your mind is racing, substitute those thoughts with the practice of a mantra that you can repeat silently or aloud. The ideal mantra can vary from person to person, but I recommend a few powerful ones to begin with (see Chapter 4 or later on in this chapter).

Secondly, keep a journal of what you are thinking about to help you know in what areas your psyche is running amok and how these thought patterns relate to your stress levels.[155] Thirdly, establish a meditation routine and try as best as you can to keep your overall practice going forward, whether it is yoga *asana*, breathing, mindfulness, etc. Lastly, consider working with someone who can guide you through this process. You deserve to invest in yourself, whether it is taking a class, joining a wellness program, working with a coach or teacher, attending a workshop or retreat, etc.

Notice how when you are engaged and fully aware in the present, your mind is focused and still. When you are walking, doing dishes, driving, etcetera, bring awareness to the thought processes going on in your mind. This monkey mind is a sign that we all have, to some degree, restlessness, inner disorder, and a lack of concentration that is an obstacle to greater tranquility and deeper wisdom. By harnessing your thought waves, you will gain clarity, ability to focus on the present, better sleep, and an increased sense of happiness and well-being.

Healing Your Consciousness

Toxins can come from elements like the food you eat or your environment. This is a reason why I emphasized in Chapter 4 the importance of a healthy diet. However, you must also minimize mental toxins. In the same way you fast to cleanse yourself of bodily toxins, you must fast from sensory impressions to give the mind relief from subtle elements or negative impressions.[156]

As you practice withdrawal of the senses, or *pratyahara*, you allow your consciousness to reach its natural state of emptiness. In this state of emptiness or vast, infinite space, you can also experience the present rather than oscillating between the past, present, and future, depending on where you decide to fixate the mind as thoughts come and go.

During this withdrawal of the senses, your mind calms down and inner thoughts arise in awareness. These thoughts can also be a source of toxicity, distraction, or confusion, especially if you attach to them and identify with them as subject, rather than as an object of awareness. For example, you may experience anger and thus think, "I am angry," rather than thinking "I perceive feelings of anger" and proceeding to let them go. To be effective at this letting go process, you must develop your intellect, awareness, and concentration.

By withdrawing from the senses and quieting the mind, you can experience these deep-rooted memories, habits, or behaviors at the surface of awareness and, if you are willing and able, let go to provide relief and deep healing. *Pratyahara* is a fasting of sensory impressions, which reduces toxic sources entering through your senses onto your field of consciousness (i.e., violent movies; news media; polluted city landscape; excessive noise; disharmonious, loud music; harmful relationships; etc.). In addition to *pratyahara*, breathing techniques, mantra, and meditation practices can help with the process of letting go and purification and balancing of consciousness.

You can help the process of healing your consciousness by enhancing your connection with nature or fine arts and music to bring in positive sources of subtle impressions into your field of awareness.[157] In addition, you can also bring the harmony and beauty of nature and art into your home or business by adding the right sensory stimuli and keeping all interactions peaceful, cordial, kind, and supportive within the structure where you live or work. This will create an environment of love, beauty, and harmony that promotes peace, happiness, and greater productivity.

As you walk, drive, or sit, try to take in as much of nature as you can, whether walking through a park, going hiking or camping, or gazing at the stars and taking in the entire breadth of the cosmos to bring into your consciousness healing energies that can shift you away from stress and illness. Therefore, balance the negative impressions with positive ones as much as you can, and eventually tip the scale in favor of mostly those of the positive kind.

If you want radiant mental and physical health, then you must feed the body and take care of it in the best way possible. Similarly, you want to take care of how you feed your mind because, if you do not, then the wrong sensory impressions create imbalance or neuroses rather than well-being and stability. You must develop the mind as you would the body by feeding it the right way, with the right sensory impressions.

Walk, talk, eat, breathe, and think in a way that is nourishing and healing for body, mind, and spirit. Again, you are the architect of your own well-being and spiritual growth. Just like whatever you put into your body will eventually lead to disease or health, your consciousness, being dynamic, fertile, and creative just like the body will change depending on what you feed it.

As a remedy to healing your consciousness, yoga recommends the reading of enlightening or inspiring books that change your perspective, elevate your spirit, and sublimate your thought waves, thereby tuning you with higher dimensions of self. Even being in the company of enlightened ones can be of great help.

These are all reasons why people go on retreats out in nature. They get to be in the company of enlightened ones who are opened minded, eat healthy meals, receive healing therapies, do many of the practices like the ones described in this book, have time to read and reflect, rest to regain balance and harmony, and heal their bodies and minds through the right sense impressions. Unfortunately, we often take our vacation time to do things that only serve to stimulate stress and inflammation more than relaxation and well-being, and give us the wrong stimuli and nutrition, both gross and subtle. We may go on a cruise, for example, and overeat unhealthy foods low in nutritional content, drink alcoholic beverages in excess, go to sleep late, listen to loud music, etc. No wonder we often need a day or two to recover after such a vacation!

Being present in the here and now makes you present and available to life's nourishment and makes life's wonders – yes, even small ones you ignore or do not notice – available to you. Bring mindfulness and energy to the present to become fully alive and deeply enriched and discover an imperturbable source of power and tranquility.

Marriage of East and West

Heed bestselling author Ken Wilber's advice when he recommends taking an integral approach to healing your psyche by not only seeking out Eastern approaches to health and well-being, but also Western approaches rooted in a solid body of data that supports the usefulness of psychotherapy, medications when needed, nutrition, etc. Do not focus only on an Eastern approach to your environment, as is emphasized in this book, which is to adapt to it and increase flexibility, but also use the Western method of changing your environment as well.

If an environment is less than ideal, the last thing you should do is just settle and accept it.

However, being adaptable is extremely useful because life can be unpredictable, and you can have moments where things happen that are out of your control. The key is to change what is predictable and constant, if less than ideal, and remain open and flexible to better adapt to changing circumstances.

If everything is changing at every moment, we must learn to be adaptable or fall prisoner to the sway of duality, the highs and lows of life, that move us away from balance and peace of mind. At the same time, we must find the source of true happiness within to remain ever calm and blissful.

Recognizing Impermanence

Recognizing and accepting the impermanence and change of life is crucial to the health of any relationship. Just like cells in your body are impermanent and your body is not the same body you even had a year ago, as many of your cells undergo endless cycles of death and birth, your partner is impermanent along with his or her love. The person you fell in love with is not the same, and you cannot expect love to wallow in the past stuck to how things were.

If you cannot expect a bouquet of flowers to remain fresh and permanent, then why expect your partner to do anything other than be impermanent? As best as you can, you must remain adaptable and flexible to evolve in harmony as the relationship with your partner matures.

Love is alive, and the love you once had is not the love you have now. It has gone through many cycles of death and rebirth, which is at the heart of the evolutionary process. The hope is that with each successive cycle, the love grows stronger, wiser, more all-embracing, and compassionate. But, for love to flourish over time, it must be fed, or it begins to lose traction, can even die, or may turn into hate.

If you consider something outside of you as permanent and attach to it, you suffer due to its natural impermanence. This is why yoga's ultimate goal is to get to the source of permanence, which is God or the True Self. Finding the True Self within yourself and then within others leads to eternal bliss, complete freedom, and true immortality.

By accepting the impermanence in others and penetrating the barriers they put forth affords you the clarity to make them truly happy. You will see everything and everyone as a continuation of your own being, and you will treat whomever or whatever with the love and respect that you give your own organism. Your family or you and your partner are a single organism and, if they suffer, you will feel it as well, and you will do what is necessary to alleviate that suffering.

Restore peace, gentleness, and kindness within yourself to be able to connect better with others. Gentleness is love and love inevitably leads to greater happiness and draws others to you. Sometimes we say that we love someone, but we do not do what is reflective of that, due to fear, confusion, or anger. At other times, due to stress we may be highly reactive and lack the requisite gentleness, compassion, and kindness that can bring together two beings.

Reconnect with the fountain of love that is your essence. Learning how to reestablish that connection is crucial. Note, however, that this should not be sought externally, but internally, within oneself. Otherwise, you will always be dependent on others for the love and peace of mind you should already possess. You should work avidly and patiently with unremitting devotion to become a fountain of love that can sustain and not drain others. By teaching others to do the same, you can then magnify this effect exponentially to heal the collective consciousness of your family or society.

Stress Hardiness

Suzanne Kobasa and Salvatore Maddi developed the concept of stress hardiness based on research that looked at groups of individuals with high stress occupations. They found that those who coped the best with substantial stressors where the ones who possessed three specific personality traits or characteristics, or the three Cs: control, commitment, and challenge.

All three need to be strongly applied in order to provide the courage and motivation to do the hard work of turning stresses into your advantage. If you do not have hardiness, do not fret, as this can be learned, though it is more easily acquired as a child from your parents.[158]

If you possess a high hardiness index, then you are more likely to put stressful life events into perspective and perceive them as less threatening and more like a challenge that is an opportunity for personal development. Due to this, you then experience stressful events in a way that will not impact your health in such a negative way. Therefore, psychological hardiness will serve a buffering effect on your health and well-being. Lots of research supports this and has been demonstrated for a variety of occupational groups, ranging from business executives to students, and even studies with fire-fighters and military who hold high stress and dangerous jobs.

Have belief and confidence in yourself, in being able to exert control over those predictable and constant events in your life that you want to change. If you doubt yourself, then you are less likely to create an environment suitable for growth and change and will likely not benefit from nor continue your practices. If you are in control, then you feel that you can more easily exert influence over your environment, that you can make things happen. Remember, however, that the control that matters is not outside of yourself, over objects, situations, or people, but comes from within.

Commit to being fully engaged in what you are doing from day to day and give any activity your best effort. Take a genuine interest in other people, develop a childlike curiosity about the world you live in, and increase your social contact by getting involved with others in activities that make a difference, matter to you, and, above all, bring you joy and fulfillment.

Challenge yourself to see change as a natural part of your life. Change is a good thing as it can afford you the opportunity for growth and development. You can get to the point of seeing stressful situations as opportunities rather than threats that you should fear or worry about. Work on your perspective, on reducing your feelings of hopelessness by increasing your sense of control. Reduce your feeling of hostility toward others or your situation. Be more optimistic, flexible, let go of the things that may seem important but often are just mere trivialities we tend to explode for due to our current state of stress, anger, or fear.

We talked about impermanence, and this also applies to stressful events. Notice how they are temporary events, and that we do not need to invest so much energy reacting to them as we should learning from them. Lastly, look for support and connection to help you deal with life's continued challenges. Remember that you are not alone. You have people around you who love you and want to help, if given a chance. If you need to, then look outside your circle for this additional help.

Other Key Psychological Traits

Cognitive flexibility and adaptability are two key traits that you should also work on developing more. Cognitive flexibility refers to your ability to recognize when something is not working and welcome a different approach. If you are too rigid, then you will be unable to try something else and will remain stuck with your current roles, habits, or behaviors that may be sabotaging your sense of freedom and peace.

Adaptability will allow you to receive and accept the unexpected, especially those events or circumstances that are difficult and currently bring you stress, pain, or sorrow. With an adaptable mindset, you will navigate more freely through any circumstance with less stress reactivity. You can learn to embrace even your darkest moments or inner turmoil with the grace and calmness that a loving mother would toward her own baby.

Allow yourself the opportunity to be where you are, to enjoy the moment. Be less judgmental, since our categorization and passing of judgments can be an obstacle toward peace and mental stillness. Therefore, work to liberate yourself from preconceptions and prejudices that reduce your connection with others. Everyone has something special to share, but sometimes it is difficult to see past all the barriers and behaviors people have learned to put in the way.

Also, do not forget to avoid judging yourself. The unseen forces of your psyche can be a major obstacle as our habits may have attracted negative ideology arising from various psychic sources. Be aware of this process as it is happening, smile when you recognize these antagonizing forces, and gently bid them farewell in your mind and replace them with enlivening, positive, and healing affirmations and ideas.

Let go and accept things as they come. Grow to accept the things you cannot change but work to gain the wisdom to recognize those that you can. Remember that, often, we have to bear what we do not like. As you grow in acceptance, you will see everything as rich, fulfilling, and leading to growth.

Trust yourself more to become more attuned with your own innate wisdom and intuition that rarely leads you astray. Do not strive to become or do anything all the time. Try to do less and focus more on being. You do not need to force yourself to be something and somewhere. Just enjoy being, for you already are perfect and beautiful, you just have not realized it yet.

Love yourself and your partner exactly as you are and he or she is, to break the attachment to your current circumstances. Have the willingness to see things as they are. Once you do, you open the door to heal yourself and your relationship. Otherwise, you will tend to remain stuck wrestling with what you do not like and never get to where you want to be.

Become more vigilant of yourself, your habits, behaviors, and thought processes. What feelings arise during particular situations? How are you reacting during stressful moments? What habits or behaviors keep showing up and how are they helping or hurting you? Are you taking ownership over those feelings or symptoms?

Remember that a key is to avoid linking the symptoms or feelings with a stance of "I-" or "mine-ness." Any feeling or symptoms is just an unfolding process and not yours to own. If you can view it in this way, you can more easily and dynamically let them go.

This is in fact what you realize very quickly during mindfulness practices. As you observe your thoughts arise, you avoid attaching to these mental formations and taking ownership over them. In this way, you can more easily let them go and return to the present moment full of awareness, focus, and stability. Do the same with moment to moment situations, feelings, or behaviors. They are also passing and momentary formations in consciousness and are not the real you, which is ever patient, calm, blissful, and free.

Pebble Meditation for Restructuring Consciousness

The Buddhist monk, Thich Nhat Hanh, made this type of meditation popular in the west. He describes this meditation in a children's version titled, "A Handful of Quiet: Happiness in Four Pebbles."

This meditation can be an excellent starter practice for anyone struggling with more advanced versions of meditation. This practice uses four distinct pebbles that represent freshness, solidity, reflection, and freedom. Small river rocks are ideal (two to three inches at most) as they are smooth and gentle to the touch.

To help identify each pebble, you can use special markers for rock painting to name each one: Flower, Mountain, Water, and Space. In addition, you can use the markers to do art on the opposite side of the words (see Appendix A).

However, this meditation alone can provide a healing tonic for our consciousness by providing us with purifying affirmations and visualizations that can eradicate negative ideology and enhance the power of our concentration. The pebbles should be treated with honor and respect, because if you do this practice correctly, you can infuse your intention into the pebbles themselves and use individual pebbles to overcome negative thought or emotional patterns, as we will describe shortly.

To begin, place the pouch with pebbles in front of you, a little to your left side. Sit, preferably on the floor or with a cushion under your seat. Make sure to focus intently on the pebble you are holding during each step, whether it is that you are gazing at them or, with eyes closed, feeling the sensations on your right palm or fingertips. If you get distracted at any moment, bring yourself back to the present and to the current meditation.

1) Flower (Freshness): Pick up the flower pebble with your left hand, place it on your right hand, close the hand, and observe or feel as you center yourself in the present and your breath. Take a few deep and slow breaths to calm your mind and get you focused. When you inhale, think: "I feel myself as a flower." When you exhale, think: "I feel fresh, beautiful, and joyful." Keep doing this for at least five minutes. When ready to move to the next pebble, place the flower pebble down in front of you and to your right.

You can visualize, during this step, an open field full of beautiful, colorful flowers inspiring bliss and joy. Feelings of beauty and bliss should abound during this meditation and you should see yourself as a radiant flower of your choice (i.e., lotus flower).

2) Mountain (Solid): Pick up the mountain pebble with your left hand, place it on your right hand, close the hand, and observe or make sure again that you are centered in the present and on your breath. When you inhale,

think: "I feel myself as a mountain." When you exhale, think: "I feel solid, strong, and stable." Again, practice for at least five minutes, and then place the mountain pebble down in front of you by the flower pebble.

During this phase, imagine your chest with a fiery mountain inside providing you with a strong grounding and warming effect. You should feel like you are anchored, comfortable, and immutable. See yourself, preferably seated in lotus posture, as strong and majestic as a mountain.

3) Water (Reflection): Now pick up the water pebble with your left hand, place it on your right hand, close the hand and remain centered and calm. When you inhale, think: "I am water." When you exhale, think: "I am reflecting, clear, and pure." Place the water pebble down in front of you when done, next to the two other pebbles.

For this pebble, you can visualize a crystal-clear lake that you can see straight through, with fish swimming and the reflection of a mountain landscape on the surface. You should reflect your True Self as it is within. A clear mind is like this lake, and we can penetrate into our consciousness to find any sadness, conflict, or obstacle that may exist. Like the image of the fish, any feeling or psychic scar can pass straight through the surface of the mind. Let this pass and leave. Smile and rejoice as they leave forever. Become tranquil and still like the water of the lake to have clear perceptions, especially those from within.

4) Space (Freedom): Finally, pick up the space pebble with the left hand, place it again on your right hand, close hand, and observe or feel as you center yourself in the present with your breath. When you inhale, think: "I feel myself as space." When you exhale, think: "I feel free, open, and infinite." Once you have repeated this cycle of breathing with affirmations for as long as you feel comfortable with, place the space pebble down in front of you, next to the rest of the pebbles, to complete the cycle.

Imagine yourself as bodiless, as if your consciousness were vast and encompassing the totality of the space around you. You feel absolutely free and happy, as you are not bound or caged in. You feel vast and light. Alternatively, as you repeat the affirmations, you can visualize that your consciousness frees itself from your body and assumes the form of a bird. You now soar free, far and wide, with no restrictions.

Notes

Repeat each pebble meditation in sync with your breath for at least five minutes (the longer the better). This meditation not only builds a strong mindfulness foundation, but also helps counteract any negative emotions or ideology we currently resonate with and that influence our self-esteem, pride, and confidence, or lack thereof. The pebbles can become charged with continued practice.

Therefore, anytime you feel angry or irritated, pick up the flower pebble and reconnect with what is beautiful and joyful about yourself with the flower meditation. If instead you feel frightened or uneasy, pick up the mountain pebble and do that meditation until those feelings subside or evaporate and you begin to feel strong, stable, and confident. If your mind feels cluttered and noisy, racing with thoughts, or you have many emotions coming up due to stress, you can pick up the water pebble and practice its associated meditation. Holding it should induce clarity and calmness, allowing you to see the inner workings of your mind that are causing this disturbance. Concentrating on the water pebble, as described above, should neutralize some of the effects of stress on the clarity of the mind by helping to tone down the noise and confusion generated. Lastly, we come to the space pebble. If you feel oppressed, trapped, unable to do what you want to, or bound and tense, as if trapped in your body unable to soar free, pick up the space pebble. The touch of the pebble can help you feel a great sense of freedom and happiness.

If practiced correctly and consistently various times per week, after a certain amount of time, depending on one's power of concentration, the pebbles can become suffused with the consciousness of the individual and, in a way, have a power of their own. At that point, the pebble alone can have the effects described in the previous paragraph without having to do a concentration exercise.

You could also share the effects built up within the pebbles with another person as well, if you think the person would benefit from the healing generated by your practice. Getting pebbles from an illumined master would indeed have a more powerful effect.

Keep the pebbles in a silken or woolen pouch to protect from electromagnetic radiation that can reduce the power embedded in the pebbles after a long period of consistent practice.

Variation

A wonderful alternative version of this meditation involves at least three additional people. Sit in a circle with knees touching and hands close to the two people seated by you. Person 1 starts with the flower pebble, while the other three sit and practice mindful breathing. Once Person 1 finishes that meditation for, let us say, a minute or two, instead of putting the rock down in front, he or she places the pebble on Person 2's left hand.

Person 1 then begins the mountain meditation, while Person 2 begins the flower meditation. This keeps cycling through until every person has at least gone once and has completed the four meditations. At any point that you find yourself without a pebble, just patiently practice mindful breathing, and remain centered and aware.

Person 1 will collect the pebbles as they come back, and places them in front him or herself to the right (unless the group wants to do additional cycles). This helps to build a sense of union and cooperation essential for spiritual development and empowers this practice with collective energy.

It is also ideal to practice with your family to build a sense of unity and cultivate moments of reflection. Children take nicely to this meditation, as they can color the pebbles and it is easy enough for them to do. Children may also want to collect pebbles or shells at the beach and use those instead for greater sense of connection to the object they will hold.

If practicing this meditation on your own, write in your journal how you felt before and after this practice to share with your partner, or to note how powerful your mind can be to reverse the effects of stress, anger, or frustration, for example. If practicing, with others (group version), each person can take time to share and reflect afterwards.

You can practice this with others as often as you like. It is ideal before dinner with family, followed by a healthy meal together trying to eat mindfully, as described previously. Before bedtime is great as well, to help calm the nerves and prime children (and parents!) for a restful night of sleep.

Mantras for Healing Consciousness

Use the following mantra if feeling overwhelmed with obstacles or lacking meaning.

Om Gum Ganapatayei Namaha.

"Om and salutations to the remover of obstacles, Ganapathi, for which Gum is the seed." Ganapathi is another name for the Hindu deity popular in India and yoga, Ganesha, who personifies union and removal of obstacles that prevent the resolution of inner conflicts.[159]

The following ancient mantra is universally practiced and considered the essence of all mantras that still, to this day, can free any seeker for spiritual enlightenment.

Om Bhu, Om Bhuvaha, Om Swaha
Om Maha, Om Janaha, Om Tapaha, Om Satyam
Om Tat Savitur Varenyam
Bhargo Devasya Dhimahi
Dhiyo Yonaha Prachodayat

"O self-effulgent Light that has given birth to the luminous planes of consciousness, who is worthy of worship and appears through the spiritual lens of the sun, illuminate our intellect."

The Gayatri Mantra is one of the most potent and healing recitations that possesses the supreme ability to help a practitioner discover enlightenment and awaken his or her consciousness at every level.[160]

Mul Mantra for Countering Negative Thoughts

Ek ong kaar, sat naam, karataa purakh, nirbho, nirvair

Akaal moorat, ajoonee, saibhang, gur prasaad, Jap!
Aad such, jugaad such, Hai bhee such, Naanak hose bhee such.
"One Creator. Truth is His name. Doer of everything. Fearless,
Revengeless, Undying, Unborn, Self-Illumined, The Guru's gift,
Meditate! True in the beginning, True through all the ages.
True even now. Oh, Nanak it is forever true."

This mantra is said to destroy whatever current fate is holding you back from your destiny. It is a root mantra from which your spiritual foundation can be built.

Practice this mantra while sitting with a straight spine. Repeat the mantra a minimum of five times, but ideally for at least five minutes. Snatam Kaur has a version where she repeats it for five minutes, if you want to listen to it and learn the sounds.[161] Davis S. Shannahoff-Khalsa suggests in a modified, shorter version of this mantra to focus with eyes closed on the vibration created against the upper palate and throughout the cranium to achieve a peaceful state of mind.[162]

Chapter 12:

Taking It to the Next Level

"The difference between ordinary and extraordinary is practice."

— Vladimir Horowitz

It Starts with You

No book or person can help you, if you do not first help yourself. You have all the tools at your disposal to make significant changes in your habits, behaviors, outlook, health, relationships, etc. You have willpower, concentration, reason, intuition, common sense, and faith. If any of those attributes are not well developed, then take the steps to develop them.

Obstacles will always be right around the corner, but do not let them deter you. In the previous chapter, I described how to overcome these obstacles with the power of your own mind and with very simple, yet effective techniques. If you need help implementing a program and sustaining it, then I am here to help.

In addition, you may already have people in your life willing to help you, including your partner. Surround yourself with or befriend any person in your life who is a role model in the areas you feel you are requiring growth. If you are lacking happiness, then look at those that smile and laugh often, and who possess a vibrant and positive outlook.

Talk more to others and be open and flexible. Do not pour all your problems on people but test the waters with anyone willing to help or at least listen. Bottling up feelings is the worst mistake we can make but finding the balance to communicate appropriately with others can be a challenge for us at times.

Mentors or inspirational figures are not right around the corner to help us find some answers, but their works are. Read more enlightening books rather than spending free time doing other activities like watching television.

Practice Makes Perfect

The most important part is to develop a disciplined practice that includes meditation in whatever form you find most helpful. Make the changes a part of your life, a habit that eventually you do not even have to think about, just like breathing. Make time for your practice. Often, we say to ourselves that we do not have the time, yet when we sit down and analyze it, we likely spend lots of time on other less fruitful activities. Your practice should be as important to you as feeding and bathing yourself.

The way you go about doing this can vary. You could join a yoga studio to start, watch videos, listen to guided recordings, or hire a meditation coach. Whatever you do to begin, the important thing is to establish a rhythm and stick to your practice. Work on being present in the moment at all times. Work on getting practice into your daily life as I mentioned in Chapter 7. Mantras or affirmations are great to integrate at any moment, while walking, driving, exercising, doing the dishes, doing breathing exercises, etc. They keep us present, grounded, and creating the right psychic space to do better work later on.

There will be a lot of reasons to not meditate. I remember how long ten minutes seemed at the beginning. However, after practicing for a year or two, one hour seemed like ten minutes and I still wanted more. You end up looking forward to those moments in deep concentration and quiescence. I equate the feeling sometimes to an awakened deep sleep state where, everything just evaporates away and only your own being, your own consciousness, is left. No stress, no worry exists, and when you have to stop practicing, many times you are left wanting more time to just be and rest in stillness.

You are so used to a mindless state of constant thinking and multitasking that sitting still and quiet can be a challenge, if not full of boredom. Yet it is not sitting still and quiet that is the problem. We do that often in the car, bus, plane, train, or sofa. See how easy it is to sit for hours because your mind is busy or stimulated. However, it can be so difficult to sit and meditate because the mind is asked to do nothing other than to observe internally, to be aware and step aside so the real you can be experienced without the noise and confusion.

Working through the Obstacles

When you sit for formal meditation practice, try to become aware of the thoughts and feelings that cross your mind. Do you feel overwhelmed by schedules, are you feeling rushed, do you feel the urge to move or do something else? Keep a journal and write down your sessions and what thoughts and feelings cross your mind when you practice meditation.

However, your mind will not be the only source of obstacles. The body can also be a source of distraction and discomfort. Resist the first urge to move and accept the discomfort to learn how to relax in this state and manage any soreness or pain better. This may translate into everyday life as you learn that you can tolerate discomfort with grace and control. If we never learn to work through pain, whether physical, mental, or emotional, we cannot react appropriately, with detachment or control.

Become aware during meditation, yoga, or body scan techniques. We can learn to remove ourselves from the domain of doing and superimposing, and instead dwell in just being and accepting to reduce the agitated thoughts and feelings or the bodily sensations of pain or muscle tension. In this way we can slowly learn to let go of these pent-up dense energies that are weighing us down and causing pain and suffering.

Cry if you feel like it, as it is cleansing and can be an antidote to stress, hypertension, and anger. Let go of the judgments and attachments that keep you bound to the reduced version of yourself that insists on condemning yourself or your situation. You are not this version of yourself that thinks you are the suffering body or mind, that you are this tiny ego trapped in a life that is less than you would have wanted or think you deserve, or that your current circumstance is out of your control. We all deserve greatness and moments of peace and serenity, but we must make it happen by first discovering the greatest gift we already possess, the True Self.

As much as possible, try to tune into your breath when you are feeling agitated or stressed, as this will bring about a state of increased relaxation, calmness, and stability. You can control the out-breath to make it longer and smoother as you mentally let out a sigh of relief and let go of the inner stir-rings that are inducing agitation. You can find a peaceful center that enhances the stability of the mind and allows you to see things clearly and calmly.

Practice catching yourself, not just during meditation, but during daily interactions or activities. In this way, you work on your practice even when not on your mat or in a quiet place at home. With time, you should integrate your practice into your daily activities to continue to bring the benefits of your practice to your moment-to-moment awareness.

You have it all right here in the now, and I know that, together, we can find it. You can systematically teach your body, mind, and spirit to develop calmness no matter what anxiety or fear is currently ruling your life at different times. These are temporary states like happiness or boredom. You can diminish these negative states and enhance those you find more positive, by reinforcing and installing habits that promote the positive ones.

Emotional pain, like physical pain, is trying to tell you something. Do not ignore these aches and pains as they will only bring further suffering. Emotional distress can be reduced, if you begin to cultivate the right habits and draw awareness to your reactions to sometimes simple situations that should not yield such an aggressive response. Emotional pain comes from your own actions or inactions, which should be under your control. You can choose to react differently, to not sit idle while something consumes you or to lash out without clarity and awareness.

If you continue to repress, ignore, exaggerate, or dramatize your emotions with little to no regulation, reflection, or awareness, you cannot yield any useful fruits or resolutions. From it, only doubt, confusion, or conflict can arise. Be mindful and not mindless. Cultivate the seedlings of healing, peace, and unity and not the weeds of pain, anger, and separation.

Breaking Away from Stress

Let's work together to make you free of stress and all its complications, rather than end up causing more serious problems to your health, in your relationships, or at work. At the very least, you deserve to be happier and enjoy the fruits of your labor with a crystal-clear mind, a healthy body, and many loving relationships all around. Your loved ones deserve to see the real you, and you do as well.

It is very easy to lose sight of who you are and say and do things you later regret. Your spouse or partner may be doing the same, reacting impulsively and mindlessly creating cycles of frustration, conflict, and despair. Thus, in many ways, this book and the program described are meant for the both of you, even for the whole family. I would even argue that a business owner would stand to benefit greatly from these practices as well (see the story of Marco in Chapter 7).

There may not be a better antidote to healing any type of relationship, whether intimate or business related, than getting to the source of the conflict, which is often related to the stress reactivity that one, or often both, share with each other. Even if there is love and patience and the relationship is not on the brink of collapse, do you not both deserve greater respect and peace and better connection through love and mutual understanding? Do you not want to reclaim what is yours from birth, which is happiness, unity, and freedom? Do your partner, friends, co-workers, and loved ones not deserve a better you? For that matter, do you not deserve the radiant, calm, powerful, confident, and beautiful person you truly are to be present all the time?

Your partner may have lost sight of what he or she fell in love with because you have chosen to project this impostor version of you. Help him or her see you again by finding yourself again and removing the many veils and projections you have superimposed over the spirit within that is beauty, love, and bliss. Over the eight weeks and beyond of your practice, you will expand your awareness to include more than just your breath. Include body sensations as they arise throughout the body, during body scanning or yoga *nidra*, for example. You may try to sense the body as a whole, listen to sounds, or finally observe the thought process itself as it streams across your mind's eye. These practices will allow you to slowly realize that you are not your body nor your thoughts.

Once this is in your field of awareness and you are fully conscious of it, then you can transcend it. The body and thoughts become mere objects in the field of awareness and not subjects, which we often take ownership over as "mine-ness" or "I-ness." Thus, they are not you, and you should not let them dictate who you are and how you feel.

You can affirm then that you are more, beyond the constrictions of space and time and everyday life. You affirm your wholeness more, you feel more complete and powerful, and thus let fewer events throw you off, allowing you to maintain stability and tranquility. I want this for you.

You can gain this freedom with practice and perseverance. Although these types of meditation practice are of lower order, it is nonetheless shown to be very powerful for healing and overcoming the effects of stress, and for gaining insights into the power our own thoughts have over us. With time, I can help you graduate to higher order meditation practices to help you to directly experience yourself as you really are, stripped down, empty, yet complete, whole, and filled with truth, love, and bliss.

Focus your energies so as to not waste them, and to be able to enter deeper states of consciousness that are tranquil and free. This in turn nourishes your body, mind, and spirit, making it easier to sustain such states and to relate better to others and to any situation that may present itself. I know that, with practice, you can carry this deep stability, peace, and freedom into your everyday life, and others will remark on the difference. Others may even remark the you seem Zen-like, relaxed, confident, or at peace.

Begin the Journey

If you have gotten to this point in the book, then at the very least, you are committed to change. To make headway in conquering stress and gaining greater freedom and joy, you must keep practicing and avoid judgments and expectations. Otherwise, you may give up altogether due to frustration or impatience. You will find that, as you practice you, will know what to do next. If you are struggling with implementing a program, reach out to me for help on Facebook, Instagram, or at ramasrootedtree.com. I will be updating the website constantly with new information, advice, online courses, seminars, workshops, retreats, programs (group and individual), etc.

To begin, commit the next eight weeks to work on integrating what is described in the previous chapters. Make sure to set aside forty-five minutes a day for at least six days per week for the next eight weeks. If you can do more, then better. Try to do some sort of practice in the morning to set you up for a better day. Experiment with times to practice that work best for you, but avoid practicing late at night, as this will make it very difficult to sustain the required awareness, energy, and concentration.

Avoid feelings of guilt when practicing. Remember that this time you are setting aside is not just for you but for others as well, as you will improve the quality of your relationship with your partner and other family members, as well as friends and co-workers. Do they not deserve a better, calmer, more vibrant you?

Eight-week Schedule

During Weeks 1 and 2, start with breathing with awareness of the inhale and exhale: five to ten minutes per sitting, at least. Bring moment-to-moment awareness as you do everyday things as much as possible. Keep a calendar as well to organize your days during the next eight weeks. Also, I suggest that you keep a journal to log feelings, realizations, etc. Practice body scanning or yoga *nidra*, likely a guided version, for thirty to forty-five minutes, if possible.

As you get to Weeks 3 and 4, consider longer sittings attending to your breath, surroundings, or body in seated meditation. In particular, increase your breathing practice to fifteen to twenty minutes. Fit in body scanning, alternating throughout the days with yoga *asana* for forty-five minutes/day.

During Weeks 5 and 6, alternate yoga with sitting meditation for the forty-five minutes. The meditation can be of your preference and can include a mantra (i.e., So Ham) or not. Integrate walking meditation, even during your daily activities. If you practice mindful walking in other scenarios (i.e., walking to work, at a park, or at the zoo), remember to allow yourself to walk a bit faster and possibly do two to three steps per inhale and two to three per exhale. While doing this faster mindful walking version, make sure to still affirm, "I am alive," "I am here," or "I am home," with pride and happiness in your heart.

By Weeks 7 and 8, you should be consistent, and your routine should be built into your everyday life. You should be doing at least forty-five minutes of practice (of your choice) every day. Hopefully, your partner and/or family member have joined in, or at least are supporting you throughout. Your physical and mental health should be significantly improved. If you are using a guided CD or online recording or video, consider weaning off it, as you should already know what to do by then. If you want to use a guided body scan, meditation, or yoga *nidra* occasionally, then do so, if it will keep you practicing. Remember, however, that other practices during the day that you fit in (i.e., during break at work) are additional and not part of the forty-five minutes described. The forty-five minutes should be for time at home that is specifically set aside for this purpose.

Throughout the eight weeks, make sure to eat a greater proportion of whole, plant-based foods and integrate some, if not most, of the supplements and healing herbs suggested. Practice mindful eating for at least one of your meals per week, if not more, and integrate the practice with your family at dinner, if applicable.

By the end, you should easily be able to fit in at least forty-five minutes of daily sitting meditation and/or yoga. At any point, feel free to practice some of the additional techniques mentioned throughout the book and on my website or social media, including those specific for certain mental and emotional states (i.e., anxiety, panic, etc.)

Beyond the Eight Weeks

After the eight weeks, continue to sit and meditate for at least 20 minutes, as this is one of the greatest gifts you can give to your body, mind, and spirit. Remember, however, that body scanning or yoga *nidra* can, when practiced correctly, be a form of meditation and can be substituted, if you feel that this is your preferred form of practice. Try at all costs to fit in even 5 minutes, in the midst of a major work deadline or a chaotic day or week, as this will keep you grounded, moving in the right direction, and countering the buildup of stress hormones.

Good times to fit in your practice are, (1) in the morning to set you up for a better, more productive day, (2) right when you get home to break up the stress patterns initiated at work and to bring you into a more balanced mindset that will benefit you and others in your home, (3) during breaks at work (if at lunchtime, practice before eating), and (4) before bed, but only if you are not too tired.

You should of course, practice yoga *asana* and read about the limbs or yoga in general, in particular about the *yamas* and *niyamas*. If you visit ramasrootedtree.com, and register your email, I can get you an advanced copy of another book with a foreword by the great yoga master Sri Dharma Mittra that is an excellent guide to the limbs, more advanced practices, and Self-Realization, the goal of yoga and of the evolutionary process. I highly recommend this book for a serious student or practitioner interested in discovering God-consciousness and taking their development to the next level and reach their greatest potential in the here and now.

Continue to eat healthily and work on integrating the suggested super-foods, healing herbs, etc. I will be posting recipes, tips, and other useful information on my website and social media as well.

Remember to be mindful of obstacles that will surface in a myriad of ways. Do not let these obstacles hinder your progress. Keep pushing forward with resolve, confidence, and mental fortitude. Smile and laugh more often to counter any negative ideology lurking in the background.

Do not fight your habitual energies, which will manifest through pervasive and intrusive thought patterns, especially during meditation. Instead, acknowledge these habitual energies with an inner smile as a current part of you that you are going to transcend. With time, effort, and even guidance from myself or someone else, these habitual and highly conditioned thought patterns will subside as concentration and willpower increase. With each passing day, greater calmness will be felt, and the mind will more easily rest, allowing you to enjoy just being.

Consider practicing with others, your partner, children, or a friend to build union and cooperation. Ask them even to please consider doing the eight-week program with you. This will improve your chances of success and of maintaining consistency. You will build collective energy that will aid this or any practice, but you must allow that energy to support and elevate you.

Practice being free in the present, not a slave of the past or the future. You can experience freedom to enjoy even the simplest of things, like brushing your teeth or combing your hair.

Being mindful and present in the here and now is a prelude to deeper practices for realizing your True Self. The mere act of being brings you closer to this sublime experience of directly witnessing the Real You.

I believe in you. You can do this. If you need to, use this book as a trusty companion, and keep coming back to it for reference or motivation.

Know that I am here to serve even beyond this book, and I suggest you visit my website or social media pages for important updates and information.

Good luck! I hope that our paths cross and I may continue to serve you! *Hari Om Tat Sat!*

— Ram

Appendix A:

Sample Practices, Alternate Versions, and Other Techniques

elow are a series of sequences and practices, mostly in illustrated format, that have been mentioned throughout book and are useful for dealing with stress, improving your breathing practices, and massaging your back, amongst other uses. In addition, I include a couple of forty five-minute routines with either therapeutic or Yin yoga postures, along with a sequence that can be done at work. If you need help learning how to do these postures, please reach out to me via social media or at ramasrootedtree.com.

How you feel and your level of energy will determine the amount of time you hold each pose. Use your best judgment and listen to your body. The times for each pose are only suggestions. If you are feeling sluggish and lethargic, that is the best time to do a more vigorous practice to elevate your energy level. When you are feeling overstimulated, scattered, or anxious, then that is when you should do a slower, more controlled or relaxing routine.

Additionally, I suggest that you do some breathing exercises to stimulate balance and concentration prior to any yoga posture sequence. Once you feel alert and stable, begin any of the following routines. Remember that *pranayama* is always a great complement to your practice.

After every routine, if time suffices, you can take some time to practice seated meditation observing breath, focusing on the space in between your eyebrows, etc. Lastly, while you are in any of these poses, refrain from letting go and falling asleep. Yes, you want to let go and relax your body, but take advantage of these poses and this time to do body scan, practice yoga *nidra* where appropriate, or concentrate on breathing or your spiritual eye area. These exercises can be moments for relaxation, but also concentration, which ultimately is what builds power and strength of will. Practicing with your eyes closed can aid in the concentration process.

45 Minutes Before Work to Energize and Increase Flexibility

Start in downward facing dog pose. Hold for thirty seconds or so before lunging with one foot forward (with control) into lizard pose (see below for two versions). Hold any of the poses for at least two to three minutes while breathing calmly and smoothly with your eyes closed and attention concentrated on areas of tension or on the space in between your eyebrows. You can do any of the poses shown below on one side first before switching to the other side, or, for each pose, do each side before moving to the next pose. I highly encourage you to practice in a dark room to enhance the relaxing effect and deepen the concentration inward.

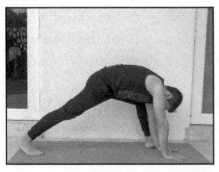

Lizard 1

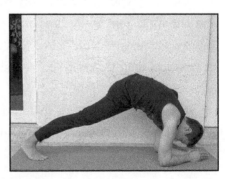

Lizard 2

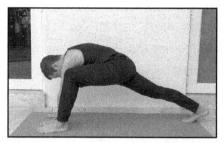

Lizard Different Side

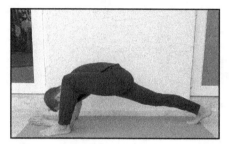

Lizard Different Side 2

After lizard pose, switch slowly to pigeon pose (two versions below).

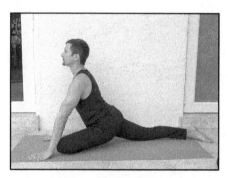

Pigeon

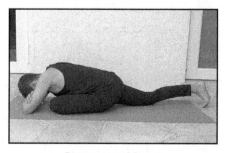

Pigeon Head Down

From pigeon you can move to half cow face pose (below). If you cannot reach your foot, do not fret. Reach wherever you can and remain still, vigilant, and as serene as possible. Keep using the breath to anchor you to the present.

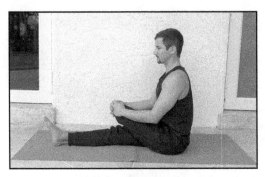

Half Cow Side View 1

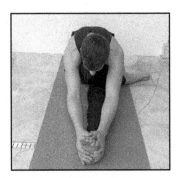

Half Cow 2

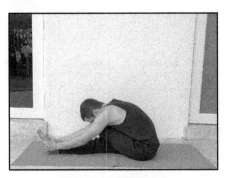

Half Cow Side View 2

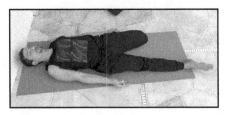

Lie Back Knee Bent

You can use support with pillows or blankets to prop you up if needed or use your elbows. The stretch may be too intense otherwise. Be mindful and possibly hold for less time avoid soreness or discomfort. However, recognize the difference between sharp pain and normal tension or soreness.

Work through the latter but avoid the former. Push yourself up with your elbows and carefully stretch your previously bent leg. Massage and shake your knee up and down to reduce some of the soreness that may linger for a few seconds afterwards (this is normal). Sit upright and bend knee. Place your ankle over your inner thigh closer to the knee than the hip. Breathe deeply with your eyes closed before leaning as far forward as possible (or with your head resting on your forearms on the floor (see below). Exert some light pressure on the space in between your eyebrows. Do both sides for three to five minutes.

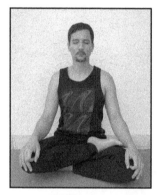
Half Lotus

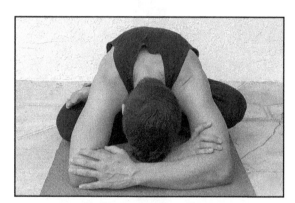
Half Lotus Head on Floor

Follow this with any of the following poses and make sure to work both sides of body, wherever applicable. Hold for at least two to three minutes and remain with your eyes closed throughout. If you cannot reach your feet, then reach to wherever you can and keep your back as straight as possible.

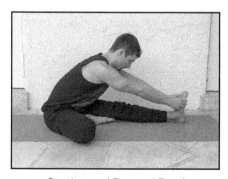
One Legged Forward Bend

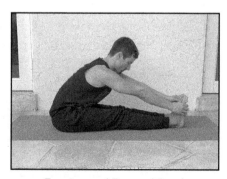
Two-Legged Forward Bend

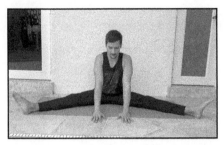

Wide Legged Forward Bend 1

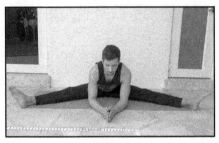

Wide Legged Forward Bend 2

You can use a pillow or prop for wide-legged forward bend (above).

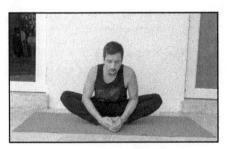

Butterfly

Your head can go all the way to floor (not illustrated). Your back should be lengthened and as straight as possible.

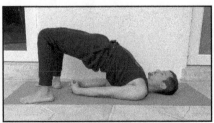

Bridge

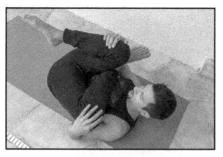

Cross Leg Knee to Head

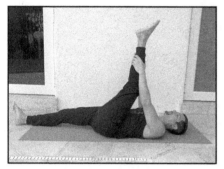

Leg Up Lying Down

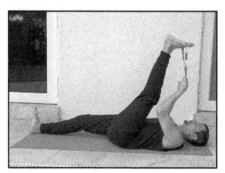

Leg Up Lying Dow with Strap

Without strap (use elbow to hold leg up)   With strap (to help keep legs straight)

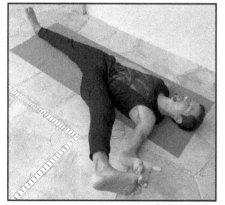

Leg to Side without Strap

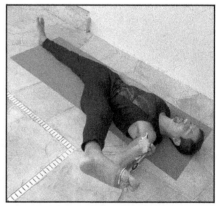

Leg to Side with Strap

45 Minutes After Work to Unwind and Rejuvenate

Once you are in a relaxed state and do not have to think about the body being twisted or stretched, then focus on the space in between your eyebrows. Use the strategies discussed earlier in the book to keep your attention grounded in the present moment.

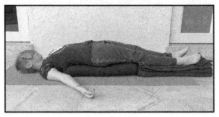

Supported Bridge

Helps correct rounded upper back (10 minutes)

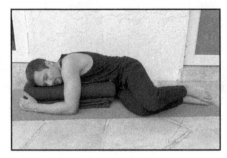

Supported Spinal Twist

5 minutes on each side

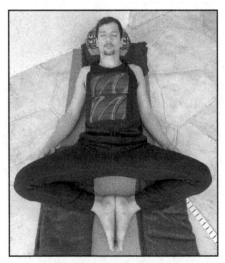

Resting Butterfly

Resting Butterfly (10 minutes)

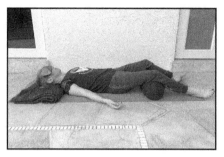

Final Relaxation High

Supported Reclining Pose (15 minutes)

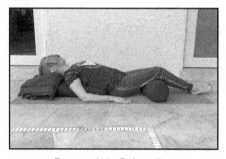

Propped Up Relaxation

You can also try this version in which you are a bit more propped up and comfortable.

Additional postures you can mix and match with (5 minutes each).

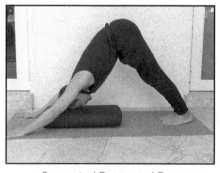

Supported Downward Dog

Supported Downward Facing Dog (5 minutes)

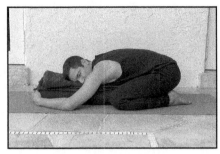

Supported Childs Pose

Supported Child's Pose (5 minutes each side)

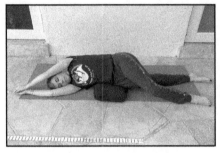

Resting Half Moon High View

Resting Halfmoon (5 minutes each side)

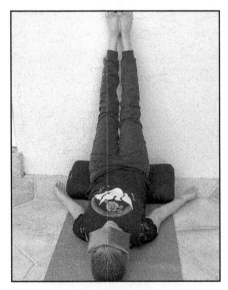

Waterfall 2

Waterfall (10 minutes)

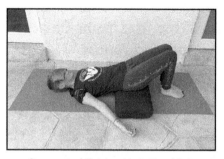

Supported Bridge Variation High

Supported Bridge Variation (5 minutes)

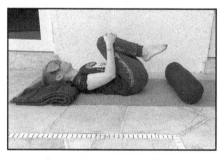

Supported Knees to Chest

Knees to Chest (5 minutes). You can do some circular movements with your legs.

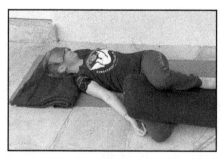

Elevated Twist

Elevate Twist (5 minutes each side)

Simple Office Practice for Upper Back Health and Increased Relaxation and Focus

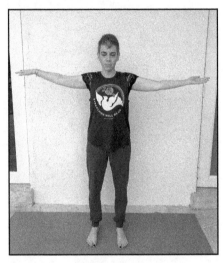

T Arms Office

Hold for two to five minutes (you eventually can reach mastery at ten minutes, although this is very difficult) to strength the upper back and reduce stress and tension on the lower back. Note that one hand faces up and the other one down.

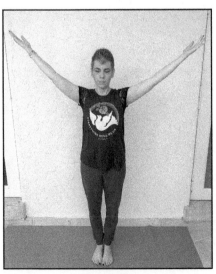

Y Arms Office

As your shoulder, arms, and upper back tire and you feel you cannot hold any longer, turn both palms facing up and raise your arms slowly from a T shape to a Y and then an I shape.

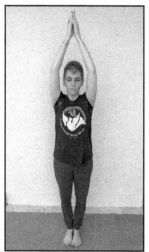
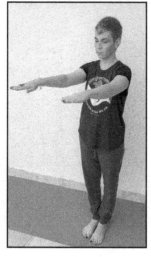
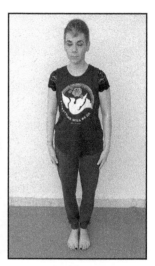

| I Arms Office | Arms In Front Office | Tadasana Office |

Finally, lower your arms slowly as you bring them into an inverted L shape and then by your sides to stand in *tadasana* or mountain pose. Slowly, reverse the movement as you lift your arms back up to an I shape and then open to Y and T shapes. Do not hold the T shape as you lower your arms back to *tadasana*. You can repeat this process two to five times. Practice this in sync with the breath by inhaling slowly as you raise arms to an I shape and exhale arms to a T shape.

Daily practice of this posture helps to correct some of the rounding of the upper back commonly seen with excessive desk work. This posture sequence will strengthen the muscles that often go dormant after many years doing desk work.

You can also sit on your heels with your back to a sofa or couch. Lean back onto a sofa chair with your hands interlaced and holding the back of your head. The rounded edge of a sofa or couch should help arch your back to counter the rounding that may have occurred over many years. You can place a pillow to prop your head. Be gentle and mindful of your upper back and areas of tension. Breathe calmly and deeply with your eyes closed and hold for two to five minutes. This position will reverse the rounding of the back and over time give you better posture and length.

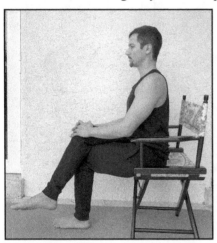
Leg Over Other No Twist Office

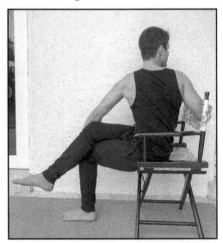
Leg Over Other Sitting Office

Cross one leg over the other with your back straight. Remain focused and breathe long and slow. On an exhale, twist gently toward the side of your top leg (right side in photo above). Take a few breaths in this position before returning back to center and repeating the process but with the other leg crossed over (left now in this sequence, see below).

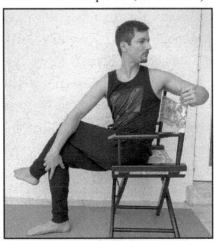
Leg Over Other Sitting Office 2

Now place both feet flat on the ground with hands over knees and inhale and arch back and look slightly upwards.

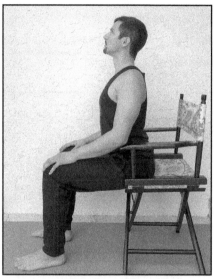

Arch Seated Office

Spine flex by arching and rounding your back. Inhale as you arch and exhale as you round the back.

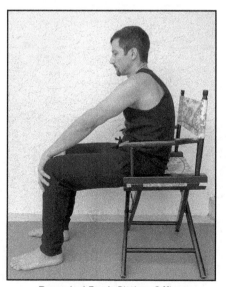

Rounded Back Sitting Office

After a couple of minutes of gently flexing your spine, place your ankle on your top leg, as shown below. You can take a moment to honor and gift your feet with a massage before continuing. Keep your back as straight as possible as you come forward on the exhale to reach to the floor if possible. If that is not possible, then rest your forearms on your legs and keep your eyes closed as you breathe deeply.

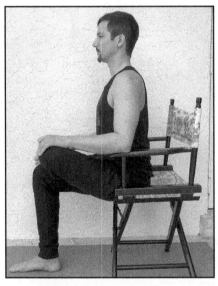

Cross Leg Straight Office

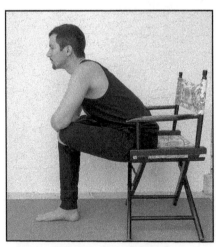

Cross Leg Lean 1 Office

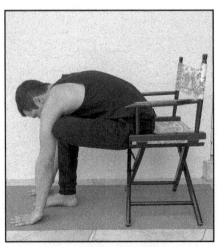

Cross Leg Lean 2 Office

After two minutes or so, come back up slowly as you inhale, making sure to lengthen your spine. Once seated upright, uncross your leg and repeat with your other ankle over your opposite leg. Sit upright again after holding for another two minutes or so and then move to the next part in the sequence.

Place both feet flat on the floor. Collect yourself and center your attention on your breath and back. On the exhale, start moving forward to reach toward the floor or your feet, with your back as straight as possible. If this is not possible, then lean forward and rest your forearms on your thighs or knees. Once you reach the floor, relax your back and let it round as you breathe into it and let your lungs lengthen the spinal cord with each inhale.

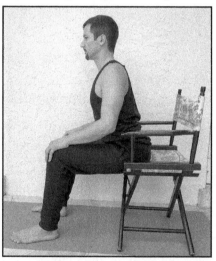

Leaning Forward Office

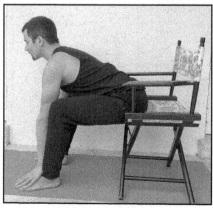

Leaning Forward 2 Office

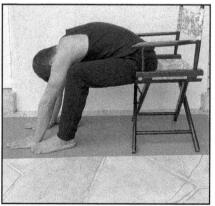

Leaning Forward 3 Office

If you can, go even deeper and breathe more fully to lengthen the spine even more.

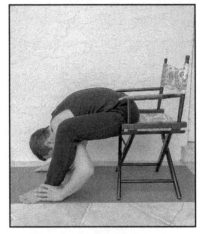

Leaning Forward 5 Office

Exhale and come back up. You want to hold the rounded posture with hands on feet or the floor for at least five minutes, if possible, as you breathe deeply using your lungs to lengthen your spine. If you do not have the five minutes, then hold for at least two minutes. The benefits of this pose are astounding.

Come into a standing forward bend to help lengthen the spine even more and counter the crunching and compacting effect of extended sitting where pressure from the seat and downward force of gravity exert a sandwich-like effect on the spinal cord and limit mobility and space between joints.

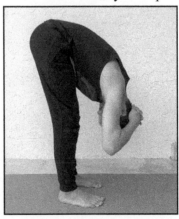

Forward Bend Standing

Rest in *savasana* or relaxation pose and do a body scan while remaining alert and using the breath as an anchor. You can place your legs on a chair to help bring blood back up the legs (this helps to diminish the appearance of varicose veins) and increase blood flow to brain centers for improved alertness and focus.

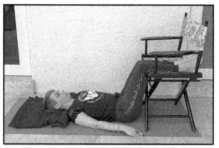

Legs on Chair Office

Sandbag Breathing

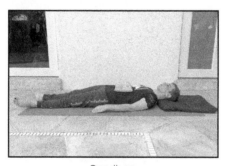

Sandbag

Makrasana or Crocodile Breathing

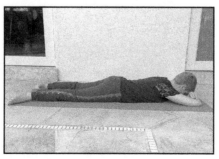

Makransana Crocodile

Suggested Seated Postures:

Padmasana or Lotus Pose

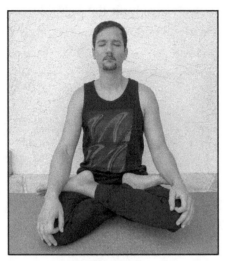

Lotus

Ardha Padmasana

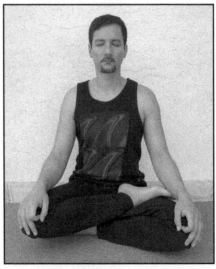

Half Lotus

Siddhasana (Easier)   Siddhasana (Harder)

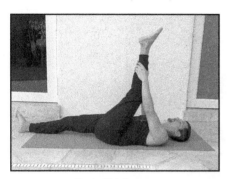 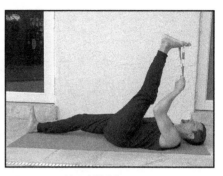

Easy Siddhasna   Hard Siddhasana

The harder version of *siddhasana* or accomplished pose requires part or most of both your feet to be tucked in between folded legs.

Sukhasana or Easy Sitting Position

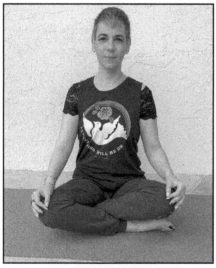

Easy Sitting

Gomukhasana or Cow Face Pose

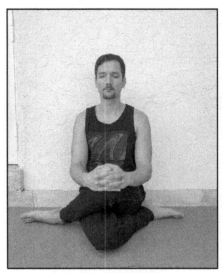

Gomukasana Cowface

Seated on Cushion

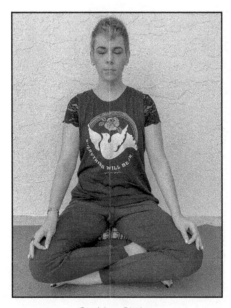

Cushion Sitting

Important Hand Gestures:

Jnana Mudra

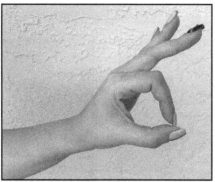

Jhana Mudra

Vishnu Mudra

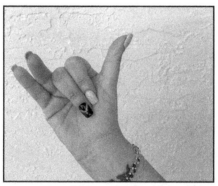

Vishnu Mudra

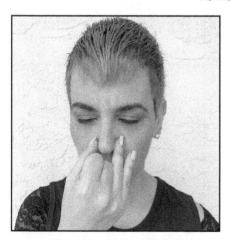

Breathing Vishnu Mudra

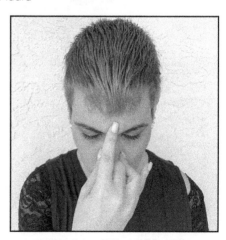

Breathing Vishnu Mudra 2

When sitting for formal meditation, you can alternatively hold hands in the gesture shown below (and in *gomukhasana*) rather than each hand in *jnana mudra* resting above each knee as has been shown previously in other images.

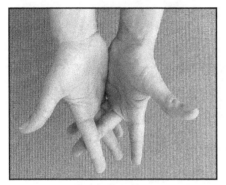

Hands Together

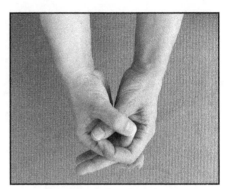

Hands Interlaced

Rocking, Rolling, and Twisting Postures:

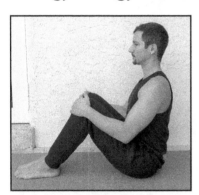

Roll Prep

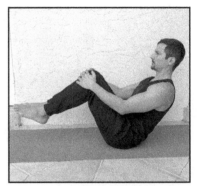

Roll 2

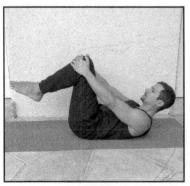

Roll 3

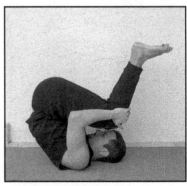

Roll 4

You can roll back and forth massaging the entire spine. Again, try to do this with eyes closed and focused on your breath. Inhale as you roll back, and exhale as come back up.

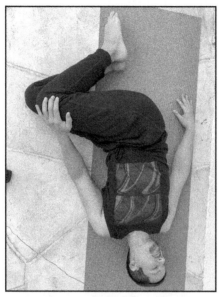

Twist 2

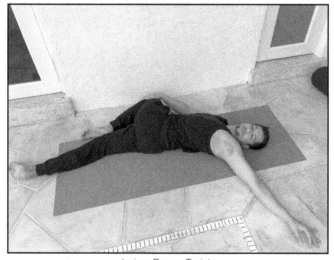

Lying Down Twist

When doing twists, please make sure to twist to both sides. Remain still with easy, deep breathing for a minute or two.

Supported Poses for Relaxation:

Supported Child's Pose

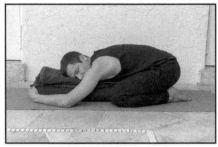

Supported Child's Pose

Supported *Titli* Asana or Butterfly Pose

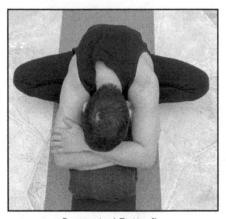

Supported Butterfly

Resting *Hamsasana* or Swan

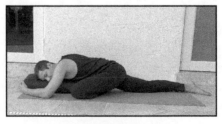

Supported Pigeon 2

Resting *Parsva bhuja dandasana* or Dragonfly

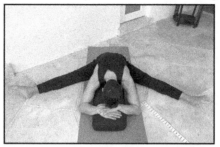

Wide-Legged Supported Forward Bend

Folded Half Lotus

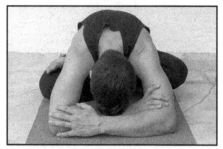

Half Lotus Head on Floor

Can also be done in lotus, if more flexible. You can exert pressure on space in between the eyebrows while in that position to stimulate your attention there.

Supported Inversions to Stimulate Alertness and Relaxation:

Supported *Adho mukha svanasana* or Downward Dog

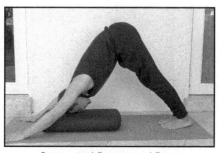

Supported Downward Dog

Inversion Preparation for Headstand (Easy version for anyone)

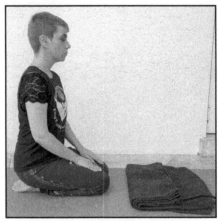

Easy Head Inversion Prep

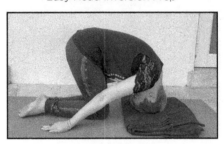

Easy Inversion

Pincha Mayurasana or Forearm Stand	*Sirsasana* or Headstand	*Salamba Sarvangasana* or Supported Shoulder Stand
Forearmstand	Headstand	Shoulderstand

NOTE: You can try the headstand or forearm stand against a wall if you are a beginner or try the preparation for headstand pose. If shoulder stand is too challenging, you can try legs up the wall (below).

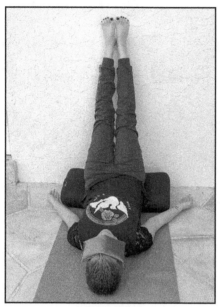

Waterfall 2

Neti Pot Use

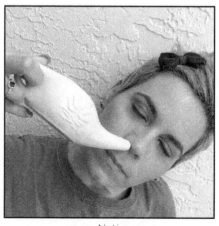

Neti

Pebbles for Meditation

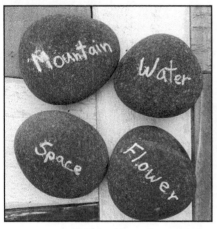

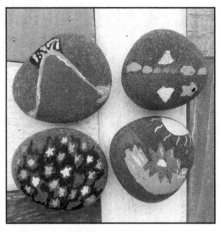

Pebbles Name   Pebbles Drawing

Appendix B:

Additional Superfoods and Healing Herbs

Below is a list of additional foods, supplements, and herbs that I recommend integrating into your diet in some way or another. All of them will help reduce oxidative stress and inflammation and enhance bodily functioning to improve your mental and physical health. Remember that you should always feed our body the right way, so you build and maintain genetic, cellular, biochemical, hormonal, and physiological well-being that you will feel at a subjective or mental level, enhance your vitality and power, and allow you to more effectively cope with stress.

Spirulina is a type of cyanobacteria or blue-green algae that is very high in nutrients (nature's multivitamin). The main antioxidant found in spirulina is phycocyanin, which gives it its blue-green color and can provide antioxidant, anti-inflammatory, and neuroprotective effects.[163,164,165] In addition, spirulina may have anti-cancer properties[166,167,168] and may enhance endurance and exercise performance.[169]

Chlorella is another nutritious algae ideal for detoxification[170,171] and enhancing the immune system.[172,173] Chlorella also contains several antioxidants, including chlorophyll, lycopene, and vitamin C, amongst a few others.[174] More importantly, chlorella may prevent DNA damage and slow down aging (telomere shortening).[175] Both spirulina and chlorella are best raw in a powder form that you can add to juices or smoothies, for example.

Kombucha Tea is a fermented tea that has been around for thousands of years. As with many of the healing remedies of ancient origins, it has a positive, holistic influence over our health. Kombucha is a great vegan source rich with probiotics that may help lower social anxiety.[176]

Being made, in part, with green tea, it may provide similar benefits. With its powerful polyphenols and acetic acid, kombucha has antioxidant and antimicrobial properties. As we have mentioned already, the polyphenols it contains give it anti-cancer properties as well. Kombucha can be made at home, but you have to know what you are doing, and thus I suggest buying one of the many different commercially available options.

Ginseng has been used for centuries as an excellent holistic therapy. The two most common types are American (panax quinquefolius) and Asian ginseng (panax ginseng). Both are considered excellent adaptogenic roots that seem to have opposed effects. The American version is more relaxing and cooling, while the Asian counterpart is stimulating and heating.[177,178] Therefore, take care when consuming these as a supplement because, depending on your mood, stress levels, or *dosha* predominance, you may benefit from one versus the other, and this could even vary by day in some cases.

Besides those differential effects, both types of ginseng, possessing ginsenosides and gintonin, have tremendous health benefits. However, unlike with many of the herbs, roots, and superfoods discussed in this book, I suggest you consult a health expert when it comes to their use, due to its cognitive and metabolic effects.

Nonetheless, fermented ginseng has been found to possess excellent antioxidant and anti-inflammatory properties.[179] Other reported benefits include enhanced working memory, decreased fatigue, anti-cancer, immune boosting effects, amongst many others. However, again the effects of each ginseng are likely distinct from each other to some extent.[180]

Camu-camu is a tropical berry often purchased in the United States in powder form added to freshly made juices or smoothies. Camu-camu has strong antioxidant and anti-inflammatory properties that lowers oxidative stress markers better than vitamin C alone.[181]

Resveratrol is a compound found in high concentration in the skins and seeds of berries (i.e., mulberries) and grapes. The most interesting finding with resveratrol is its anti-aging properties. In a study in the prestigious journal Nature, resveratrol increased lifespan in yeasts by seventy percent, likely through a mechanism involving increased DNA stability.[182] Similar results have been found in a few other species, though studies with humans are lacking.

Another interesting application of resveratrol supplementation is its possible role as a neuro-protector and as a treatment or prevention of neurodegenerative conditions such as Alzheimer's disease.[183,184,185] Lastly, resveratrol may suppress cancer tumor growth by preventing cell replication and altering gene expression.[186,187]

Resveratrol is often taken as a supplement in capsule form, since the amounts found in berries, grapes, or wine may not be sufficiently high enough for a positive effect. However, researchers are not convinced we can make use of the supplemental versions of resveratrol. Thus, for now, it may be best just to consume the foods that contain it for whatever benefits it may provide.

Mint is the name given to over a dozen plants. Often thought of mainly as providing a refreshing flavor and sensation, mint is actually rich in nutrients, including vitamin A and a number of antioxidants. Mint is very beneficial for the digestive system, as it is helpful as an adjunct treatment for irritable bowel syndrome, which is often the result of chronic stress, and also helps with upset stomach and indigestion. The scent of its oil can increase alertness and decrease anxiety and fatigue that is often seen with stress.[188] Mint can be ingested as a tea or the leaves juiced, blended, or eaten in a salad, or its oil can be heated for a delightful aromatherapy with significant cognitive effects.

Cacao powder is one of the richest sources of polyphenols (flavanols), which we described previously as having strong antioxidant and anti-inflammatory effects. However, what you want is a raw source (likely in powder form) because the more processed versions have diminished polyphenol content (up to sixty percent). As we know, polyphenols have many benefits, and thus flavanols found in cacao are no exception. Effects range from cancer prevention to enhanced brain function by increasing blood supply to the brain, as it can cause vasodilation.[189,190] The latter effect makes flavanols in cacao an adjunct treatment for high blood pressure.[191,192] In addition, high-polyphenol cacao enhances mood in humans possibly by reducing stress levels.[193,194]

Wheat Germ is the mineral- and vitamin-rich part of the wheat kernel. It is in essence the embryo of the plant and thus the most nutritious part. Unfortunately, we often do not consume it, as it is lost during the processing of most wheat products. Although data is still lacking, wheat germ should be an integral part of your diet, as it may help reduce the risk of cardiovascular disease by lowering cholesterol. In addition, avemar, a fermented wheat germ extract, has anti-inflammatory effects, making it an option to consider as an adjunct therapy for arthritis.[195,196] You can add wheat germ, either toasted or raw, to smoothies, cereals, and baked goods, or as a topping on a number of dishes or desserts.

Hemp Seeds come from the *Cannibis sativa* plant. Yes, the same plant as marijuana, but a different variety that only contains trace, insignificant amounts of the plant's psychoactive component, tetrahydrocannabinol. These seeds are a must have in any diet, especially a vegan, whole, plant-based one, as these seeds are incredibly nutritious and rich in the healthiest of fats, the omega fatty acids, that are essential for your brain development and function, and as an adjunct treatment for mental illness.[197] They are also a great source of high-quality protein that is non-toxic and easy to digest. Lastly, hemp seeds are a rich source of antioxidants and important minerals. You should ideally consume these seeds raw and whole, and add them to smoothies, cereals, and baked goods.

Cannabidiol: The marvelous hemp plant also possesses a non-psycho-active oil, called cannabidiol (CBD), which is often diluted in hemp seed oil and added to food, taken as a supplement, or applied topically. This oil has been growing in popularity worldwide and its benefits are slowly being supported by a growing body of scientific evidence. In addition, CBD is tolerated well with minimal side effects.[198] Reports suggest it is effective in reducing pain,[199] inflammation,[200] addiction,[201] and anxiety,[202] and treating insomnia,[203] amongst various other uses. However, make sure the product is of high quality, organic, and containing full-spectrum oil, which has other phytocannabinoids working synergistically with cannabidiol to boost its health effects.

Ideally, you should take the oil without heating it by adding the suggested dosage (i.e., ten drops in the morning and evening) under the tongue for better health results, as vaporizing the oil requires heating and damages or oxidizes the phytocannabinoids further. For the best quality products, look for CBD oils that have 500 to 750 mg shown to be within the range of doses having clinical effects (typically 600 mg).[204,205]

Quinoa, the mother of all grains, is another high protein, gluten-free option, and one of the few plants with all nine essential amino acids. Like hemp seeds, it is highly nutritious with lots of minerals, vitamins, and antioxidants. This super grain even contains flavonoids, like kaempferol and quercetin, which we have mentioned before provides many health benefits (i.e., anti-inflammatory, anti-cancer, and anti-depressant effects). Quinoa is very easy to cook and incorporate into your diet, as it goes well with many foods. You can add it to a tasty kale salad or substitute it for rice.

Chia Seeds are a low-calorie superfood packing in lots of nutrition, antioxidants, protein, omega-3 fatty acids, and soluble fiber. Add these seeds to smoothies, drinks, cereals, and baked goods, or make them into pudding with your favorite nut milk, banana, and cacao.

Flax Seeds are another emerging superfood with many health-protective effects. Flax seeds contain plenty of protein, fiber, and omega fatty acids, in addition to a variety of vitamins and minerals. One of flax's most remarkable features is that it contains enormous amount of lignans, a compound found in plants with antioxidant properties. Enjoy raw flax seeds similarly to the seeds previously mentioned.

Oats are one of the healthiest whole-grains on the planet. Oat groats are the most unprocessed, and thus the healthiest. However, they take a long time to cook, and therefore most people prefer steel-cut or rolled oats. Oats a great source of the powerful fiber beta-glucan, which can help you lower cholesterol, treat diabetes, and lose weight.[206,207,208] If you consume whole oats, then you are getting a food source rich in polyphenols and the anti-inflammatory antioxidants, called avenanthramides. Eat your oats as a porridge or add them to smoothies or baked goods.

Pomegranates may very well be the king of all fruits, a Zen fruit when it comes to mindful eating, as separating and eating the seeds cannot be rushed and therefore the fruit must be eaten slowly, with great care, focus, and awareness. I highly suggest that you practice eating this fruit mindfully, when in season, as often as you can afford.

Pomegranates come from a shrub that produces a red fruit with many delicious and tart seeds surrounded by a bitter, inedible skin. Even a single cup of this fruit is highly nutritious and contains plenty of protein, vitamins, and minerals. Pomegranates contain two powerful medicinal compounds, punicalagins and punicic acid. Punicalagins are some of the most potent antioxidants in nature. However, to get higher content of punicalagins and antioxidant content, you will need an extract of the whole fruit with peel. You find punicic acid in the seed as its main fatty acid. There are gel capsules that contain all of these key components.

I mentioned in Chapter 4 that chronic inflammation is a problem you cannot ignore, as it can work synergistically with chronic stress to exacerbate many common western diseases, including cancer, type-2 diabetes, Alzheimer's disease, etc. Pomegranates, with their punicalagins, can lower inflammatory and cancer markers[209,210] and help fight Alzheimer's disease.[211]

As with any fruit, pomegranates should be eaten fresh, never in pre-made juice bottles. Additionally, I suggest a daily soft gel of whole fruit, seed, and flower to supplement.

Berries, such as goji berries, acai, and black-, blue-, straw-, and rasp-berries, have one of the highest concentrations of antioxidants of the commonly consumed fruits, after the levels found in fresh pomegranates. Berries are very nutritious, high in fiber and antioxidants, help control sugar levels, etc. We already know the importance of antioxidants in fighting oxi-dative stress and inflammation in our body and protecting against cancer. In addition, do not forget that consuming foods that reduce stress and increase energy enhances our feelings of well-being, as has been shown for goji berries.[212] Add them to salads, cereals, smoothies, or eat them on their own.

Schisandra is a vine plant that bears adaptogenic berries. These are not typical berries, as they are not commonly eaten as food. However, they possess a number of compounds that provide significant health benefits, including stress and anxiety reduction, antidepressant effects, and anti-in-flammatory and neuroprotective effects. This is usually taken as a supple-ment in multiple ways (powder, pills, extracts, etc.).

Exotic fruits that I recommend and that have many of the benefits and nutrition that we have listed for other superfoods are: (1) Baobab, a citrus-like flavored large fruit, (2) jackfruit, one of the largest tree-borne fruits in the world and with superb flesh for delicious vegan dishes, and (3) lychee, a sweet fruit with oligonol that may help reduce visceral fat.

Raw nuts, seeds, or legumes, especially soaked or sprouted, are a valuable addition to your diet, as they will provide you with lots of protein, omega-3 fatty acids, fiber, vitamins, and minerals. In particular, consider increasing your intake of lentils, which contain one of the highest sources of antioxidants and may help boost mood and lower anxiety. These legumes are also extremely versatile to be used in many ways in the kitchen, are delicious, high in protein and key minerals, and also very affordable.

Acknowledgements

F irstly, I would like to thank my parents for raising me to be a free thinker, unbound and unencumbered by dogma or preconceptions. It has been a long journey to this point, and I would like to honor the people, especially the women, who were instrumental in helping this book and other books in the future see the light of day and for this movement to start. Brave, strong, and kindhearted women are at the core of the humankind's ascent back to its greatness. Writing this book without honoring some of them would be a dishonor and a disservice.

To Dr. Doris Ramirez-Soto, professor of Chemistry at the University of Puerto Rico, who first noticed the creativity within me, and helped pave the way for my acceptance into one of the top Neuroscience doctorate programs in the world.

To Dr. Amy F.T. Arnsten, who showed me the art of storytelling to help bring even the most complex of ideas into the minds and hearts of anyone who would listen. She is a fantastic leader who patiently and lovingly nurtured my growth as a scientist, writer, and speaker.

I would like to give thanks as well to my loving and loyal wife Norma.

I know I would not be where I am now, if it were not for her undying support, advice, and love. She is the foundation upon which our house can stand firm. She has provided many ideas and suggestions along the way and has bravely pursued the process described in this book to help demonstrate firsthand its usefulness, practicality, and immense healing potential.

I would also like to thank Dr. Angela E. Lauria and her fabulous team at Author Incubator and Difference Press. In particular, I would like to thank Dr. Lauria for being such a bright spirit always making herself available to help other become agents of service and truth in alignment with their destiny and the universe as a whole. Her help throughout this book has not gone unnoticed and is greatly appreciated. She helped to me to realize how to marry a servant's heart with a business model that could touch many a life and make a difference.

I would also like to thank Ora North, Cheyenne Giesecke, and Bethany Davis. Ora was incredibly helpful and patient offering many suggestions and edits during the making of this book. Cheyenne was always so kind to offer guidance or help I may have needed along the way. Bethany was the managing editor who kindly and graciously offered her service and expertise to enhance the readability and appeal of book.

To the Morgan James Publishing team: Special thanks to David Hancock, CEO & Founder for believing in me and my message. To my Author Relations Manager, Gayle West, thanks for making the process seamless and easy. Many more thanks to everyone else, but especially Jim Howard, Bethany Marshall, and Nickcole Watkins.

Finally, I would like to thank the entire community of writers at the Author's Way on Facebook for their support and generosity. They helped make the writing of this book a much smoother and enjoyable process.

Thank You

Thank you so much for reading this book. The fact that you have gotten to this point tells me that you are committed to mastering the art of living a stress-free and healthy life that can enrich your relationships and even your business. You are ready to take this to the next level. You are ready to experience the Real You, happy, vibrant, and free.

To support you through this process and to facilitate your progress through the program, visit me at www.ramasrootedtree.com to set-up a FREE consultation and for FREE recordings of all mantras in this book. In addition, I suggest you visit me on social media (#ramasrootedtree) to ask me any questions or visit my blog for monthly updates of events, recipes, research finding, etc. To get the most benefit, I highly suggest that you consider one of our life-changing programs, especially our DNA Reprogramming Blueprint, where you can get to work with me and attend my annual live events. *Hari Om Tat Sat!*

Love and Divine Grace always,

Ram

Miami FL, 2019

About the Author

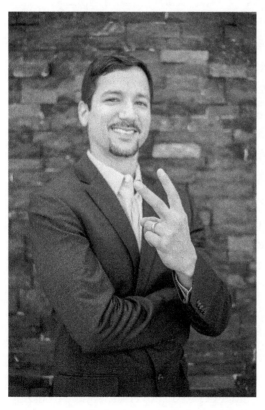

Dr. Brian P. Ramos, affectionately known as Ram by his closest students, earned his bachelor's degree in clinical microbiology from the University of Puerto Rico – Mayaguez in 1999 before obtaining his Ph.D. in Neurobiology from Yale University in 2005. Dr. Ramos is the author of numerous publications in the area of neuroscience and molecular psychiatry with a special interest in stress-related disorders, cognitive enhancement, aging, and behavior.

He is a Dharma Mittra Yoga and Therapeutic Yoga certified instructor and certified to teach yoga for children and adolescents with or without neurodevelopmental issues. His approach to yoga is integral and conducive to higher states of consciousness; deep, conscious relaxation; radiant health and vitality; and powerful genetic transformations.

He has been the President and owner of Miami Healthy You Vending since 2016 as part of an effort to bring more wellness options to corporations looking to improve the mental and physical health of their employees. In 2018, he founded Rama's Rooted Tree Healing Center to bring true healing and transformational growth into higher dimensions of consciousness through his unique and conscious DNA Reprogramming Blueprint that is part of his stress reduction, healing, and self-realization programs.

From 1995-1999, Dr. Ramos worked at a nonprofit Spiritist center called Instituto de Cultura Espirita Renacimiento, led by Dr. Flavio Acaron, where he helped to heal many a person suffering from a variety of physical, mental, and spiritual conditions. During his work there, he saw the potential inherent in humans, the power of latent psychic abilities, the vast dimensions of consciousness untapped or unrealized by most, and the need to improve mental health and chronic care.

During his many studies, Dr. Ramos aimed to learn about the nervous system and how we are connected, as infinite spirits, to the body through our nervous and endocrine networks and genetic programs. During graduate school and even after obtaining a Ph.D., Dr. Ramos immersed himself for years in the study of the effects of stress on the nervous and endocrine systems. In addition, he studied for many years how stress and other mental states influence our health as our body ages and how it changes our gene expression for better or worse.

In his early twenties, Dr. Ramos rediscovered Yoga and Ayurveda, which provided him with many of the adjunct therapies and techniques described in this book. He pursued the path of self-realization and introspection through advanced yogic practices to discover the source of happiness and peace, which is at the core of our being.

Dr. Ramos, along with Guillermo Yorio, developed a multimedia tool-kit titled *Getting to Know and Overcoming Stress* (in Spanish) at <u>solulife.com</u>. That is when he first began to develop the practices and techniques for application to stress reduction and management described in this book.

Dr. Ramos is a compassionate individual who lives to serve others no matter what their background or their difficulties. He is an assiduous student with vast breadth of knowledge not only in his area of specialty, but also including, amongst other disciplines, medicine, nutrition, health, Ayurveda, Spiritism, mediumship, psychic healing, meditation, and consciousness research.

Dr. Ramos lives with his wife and children in Miami Lakes, Florida.

Endnotes

1   https://abcnews.go.com/US/superhero-woman-lifts-car-off-dad/story?id=16907591
2   https://tucson.com/news/local/crime/article_e7f04bbd-309b-5c7e-808d-1907d91517ac.html
3   https://www.theglobeandmail.com/news/national/protective-mother-wrestles-lost-polar-bear/article703773
4   Gordan R., Gwathmey, J.K., and Xie, L-H. Autonomic and endocrine control of cardiovascular function. World J Cardiol. 2015; 204-214.
5   Costa K.M., et al. Evolution and physiology of neural oxygen sensing. Front Physiol. 2014; 302.
6   Messina, G., et al. Autonomic nervous system in control of energy balance and body weight: personal contributions. Neurol Res Int. 2013; 2013:639280. doi: 10.1155/2013/639280. Epub 2013.
7   Guyenet, P.G. The sympathetic control of blood pressure. Nat Rev Neurosci. 2006; 7(5): 335-46.
8   Jacobs, G.D. Clinical applications of the relaxation response and mind-body interventions. J Altern Complement Med. 2001; 7 Suppl 1:S93-101.

9   https://www.scientia.global/professor-amy-arnsten-staying-control-prefrontal-cortex-helps-us-human/

10 Arnsten, A.F.T. Stress signaling pathways that impair prefrontal cortex structure and function. Nat Rev Neurosci. 2009; 10(6): 410-422

11 Lu, N.Z., Wardell, S.E., Burnstein, K.L., Defranco, D., Fuller, P.J., Giguere, V., Hochberg, R.B., McKay, L., Renoir, J.M., Weigel, N.L., Wilson, E.M., McDonnell, D.P., Cidlowski, J.A. International Union of Pharmacology. LXV. The pharmacology and classification of the nuclear receptor superfamily: glucocorticoid, mineralocorticoid, progesterone, and androgen receptors. Pharmacol Revl. 2006; 58 (4): 782–97.

12 Cadet, J.L., Brannock, C., Jayanthi, S., Krasnova, I.N. Transcriptional and Epigenetic Substrates of Methamphetamine Addiction and Withdrawal: Evidence from a Long-Access Self-Administration Model in the Rat. Mol Neurobiol. 2014; Jun 18. Epub.

13 Arnsten, A.F.T. The biology of being frazzled. Science. 1998; 280(5370): 1711-12.

14 Arnsten, A.F.T. Catecholamine influences on the dorsolateral prefrontal cortical networks. Biol Psychiatry. 2011; 69(12):e89-99. Doi: 10.1016/j.biopsych.2011.01.027. Epub 2011. Apr 13. Review.

15 Lu, N.Z., Wardell, S.E., Burnstein, K.L., Defranco, D., Fuller, P.J., Giguere, V., Hochberg, R.B., McKay, L., Renoir, J.M., Weigel, N.L., Wilson, E.M., McDonnell, D.P., Cidlowski, J.A. International Union of Pharmacology. LXV. The pharmacology and classification of the nuclear receptor superfamily: glucocorticoid, mineralocorticoid, progesterone, and androgen receptors. Pharmacol Revl. 2006; 58 (4): 782–97.

16 Rhen, T. and Cidlowski, J.A. Anti-inflammatory action of glucocorticoids: new mechanisms for old drugs. N. Engl. J. Med. 2005; 353 (16): 1711–23.

17 Karssen, A.M., Her S, Li, J.Z., Patel, P.D., Meng, F., Bunney, W.E. Jr, Jones, E.G., Watson, S.J., Akil, H., Myers, R.M., Schatzberg, A.F., Lyons, D.M. Stress-induced changes in primate prefrontal profiles of

gene expression. Mol Psychiatry. 12(12):1089-102. Epub 2007; Sep 25. Review.

18   Wellman, C.L. Dendritic reorganization in pyramidal neurons in medial prefrontal cortex after chronic corticosterone administration. J Neurobiol. 2001; 49(3):245-53.

19   De Feo, P., et al. Contribution of cortisol to glucose counterregulation in humans. Amer J of Physiol Endocrinol and Metabol. 1989; Vol. 257. E35-E42.

20   Rizza, R.A., Mandarino, L.J., Gerich, J.E. Cortisol-induced insulin resistance in man: impaired suppression of glucose production and stimulation of glucose utilization due to a postreceptor defect of insulin action. J Clin Endocrinol Metab. 1982; 54(1):131-8.

21   Okabayshi, Y., et al. Mechanisms of insulin-induced insulin-receptor downregulation: Decrease of Receptor biosynthesis and mRNA levels. 1989; 38(2): 182-187.

22   Chiodini, I., Adda, G., Scillitani, A., Coletti, F., Morelli, V., Di Lembo, S., Epaminonda, P., Masserini, B., Beck-Peccoz, P., et al. Cortisol secretion in patients with type 2 diabetes: relationship with chronic complications. Diabetes Care. 2007; 30(1):83-8.

23   Coutinho, A.E. and Chapman, K.E. The anti-inflammatory and immunosuppressive effects of glucocorticoids, recent developments and mechanistic insights. Mol Cell Endocrinol. 2011; 335(1): 2–13.

24   Weinrib, A.Z., Sephton, S.E., Degeest, K., Penedo, F., Bender, D., Zimmerman, B., Kirschbaum, C., Sood, A.K., Lubaroff, D.M., Lutgendorf, S.K. Diurnal cortisol dysregulation, functional disability, and depression in women with ovarian cancer. Cancer. 2010; 116(18):4410-9.

25   https://www.medicalnewstoday.com/releases/197877.php

26   Finterwald C. and Alberini C.M. Stress and glucocorticoid receptor-dependent mechanisms in long-term memory: from adaptive responses to psychopathologies. Neurobiol Learn Mem. 2014; 17-29. Doi: 10.1016/j.nlm.2013.09.017. Epub 2013 Oct 7.

27 Possessing the luminous, spiritual quality or inducing a change in us toward balance, harmony, health, serenity, and peace.

28 Campbell, T.C. and Campbell, T.M. The China Study: Revised and expanded edition: The most comprehensive study of nutrition ever conducted and the startling implications for diet, weight-loss, and long-term health. BenBella Books. 2016.

29 LaChance, L.R. and Ramsey, D. Antidepressant foods: An evidenced-based nutrient profiling system for depression. World J Psychiatr. 2018; 8(3): 97-104.

30 Schinasi, L. and Leon, M.E. Non-Hodgkin lymphoma and occupational exposure to agricultural pesticide chemical groups and active ingredients: a systematic review and meta-analysis. Int J Environ Res Public Health. 2014; 11(4): 4449-4527.

31 Torretta, V., et al. Critical review of the effects of glyphosate exposure to the environment and humans through the food supply chain. Sustainability. 2018; 10: 950.

32 https://www.reuters.com/article/us-monsanto-cancer-lawsuit/monsanto-ordered-to-pay-289-million-in-worlds-first-roundup-cancer-trial-idUSKBN1KV2HB

33 Liu, Y-Z, Wang, Y-X, and Jiang, C-L. Inflammation: The common pathway of stress-related diseases. Front Hum Neurosci. 2017; 11: 316.

34 Kiecolt-Glaser, J.K., et al. Omega-3 supplementation lowers inflammation and anxiety in medical students: a randomized trial. Brian Behav Immun. 2011; 25(8): 1725-34.

35 Sah, A.K., Vijaysimha, M., and Mahamood, M. The tulsi, queen of green medicines: Biochemistry and pathophysiology – A Review. Int J Pharm. 2018; 50(2): 106-114.

36 Cohen, M.M. Tulsi – Ocimum sanctum: A herb for all reasons. J Ayurveda Integr Med. 2014; 5(4): 251-259.

37 Nagababu, E., et al. Assessment of antioxidant activity of eugenol in vitro and in vivo. Methods Mol Biol. 2010; 610: 165-80.

38   Noshahr, S., et al. Protective effects of Withania somnifera root on inflammatory markers and insulin resistance in fructose-fed rats. Rep Biochem Mol Biol. 2015; 3(2): 62-7.

39   Khan, M.A., et al. Effect of Withania somnifera (Ashwagandha) root extract on amelioration of oxidative stress and autoantibodies production in collagen-induced arthritic rats. J Complementary Integr Med. 2015; 12(2): 117-25.

40   Auddy, B., et al. A standardized Withania somnifera extract significantly reduces stress-related parameters in chronically stressed humans: A double-blind, randomized, placebo-controlled study. 2008; 11(1): 50-56.

41   Chandrasekhar, K. Kapoor, J., and Anishetty, S. A prospective, randomized double-blind, placebo-controlled study of safety and efficacy of a high-concentration full spectrum extract of ashwagandha root in reducing stress and anxiety in adults. Indian J Psychol Med. 2012; 34(3): 255-62.

42   Choudary, D., Bhattacharyya, S., and Bose, S. Efficacy and safety of Ashwagandha (Withania somnifera (L.) Dunal) root extract in improving memory and cognitive functions. J Diet Suppl. 2017; 14(6): 599-612.

43   Pingali, U., Pilli, R., and Fatima, N. Effects of standardized aqueous extract of Withania somnifera on tests of cognitive and psychomotor performance in healthy human participants. Pharmacognosy Res. 2014; 6(1): 12-8.

44   Flavonoid with antioxidant effects that helps to protect the brain and reduce the risk of cancer, heart disease, and stroke.

45   Mirjalili, M.H., et al. Steroidal lactones from Withania somnifera, an ancient plant for novel medicine. Molecules. 2009; 14(7): 2373-93.

46   Gorelick, J., et al. Hypoglycemic activity of withalonides and elucidated Withania somnifera. Phytochemistry. 2015; 116: 283-289.

47   Andallu, B. and Radhika, B. Hypoglycemic, diuretic, and hypocholesterolemic effect of winter cherry (Withania somnifera, dunal) root. Indian J Exp Biol. 2000; 38(6): 607-9.

48 Vyas, A.R. and Singh, S.V. Molecular targets and mechanisms of cancer prevention and treatment by withaferin a, a naturally occurring steroidal lactone. AAPS J/ 2014; 16(1): 1-10.

49 Kakar, S.S., et al. Withaferin a alone and in combination with cisplatin suppresses growth and metastasis of ovarian cancer by targeting putative cancer stem cells. PLoS One. 2014; 9(9): e107596.

50 Candelario, M., et al. Direct evidence for GABAergic activity of Withania somnifera on mammalian ionotropic GABAA and GABAp receptors. J Ethnopharmacol. 2015; 171: 264-72.

51 Andrade, C., et al. A double-blind, placebo-controlled evaluation of the anxiolytic efficacy of an ethanolic extract of Withania somnifera. Indian J Psychiatry. 2000; 42(3): 295-301.

52 These are the most potent curcumin extracts on the market and two hundred and fifty times more potent than regular curcumin.

53 Shoba, G., et al. Influence of piperine on the pharmacokinetics of curcumin in animals and human volunteers. Planta Med. 1998; 64(4): 353-6.

54 Jurenka, J.S. Anti-inflammatory properties of curcumin, a major constituent of Curcuma longa: a review of preclinical and clinical research. Altern Med Rev. 2009; 14(2): 141-53.

55 Takada, Y, et al. Nonsteroidal anti-inflammatory agents differ in their ability to suppress NF-kappaB activation, inhibition of expression of cyclooxygenase-2 and cyclin D1, and abrogation of tumor cell proliferation. Oncogene. 2004; 23(57): 9247-58.

56 Menon, V.P. and Sudheer, A.R. Antioxidant and anti-inflammatory properties of curcumin. Adv Exp Med Biol. 2007; 595: 105-25.

57 Barclay, L.R., et al. On the antioxidant mechanism of curcumin: classical methods needed to determine antioxidant mechanism and activity. Org Lett. 2000; 2(18): 2841-3.

58 Biswas, S.K., et al. Curcumin induces glutathione biosynthesis and inhibits NF-kappaB activation and interleukin-8 release in alveolar epithelial cells: mechanism of free radical scavenging activity. Antioxid Redox Signal. 2005; 7(1-2): 32-41.

59 Agarwal, R., Goel, S.K., and Behari, J.R. Detoxification and antioxidant effects of curcumin in rats experimentally exposed to mercury. J Appl Toxicol. 2010; 30(5): 457-468.

60 Chandran, B. and Goel, A. A randomized, pilot study to assess the efficacy and safety of curcumin in patients with active rheumatoid arthritis. Phytother Res. 2012; 26(11): 1719-25.

61 Sikora, E., Scapagnini, G., and Barbagallo, M. Curcumin, inflammation, ageing, and age-related diseases. Immun Ageing. 2010; 7(1): 1.

62 Sanmukhani, J., et al. Efficacy and safety of curcumin in major depressive disorder: a randomized controlled trial. Phytother Res. 2014; 28(4):579-85.

63 Kulkarni, S.K., Bhutani, M.K., and Bishnoi, M. Antidepressant activity of curcumin: involvement of serotonin and dopamine systems. Psychopharm. 2008; 201:435.

64 Xu, Y., et al. The effects of curcumin on depressive-like behaviors in mice. Eur J of Pharmacol. 2005; 518(1): 40-46.

65 Aggarwal, B.B., Kumar, A., and Bharti, A.C. Anticancer potential of curcumin: preclinical and clinical studies. Anticancer Res. 2003; 23(1A): 363-98.

66 Pole, Sebastian. Ayurvedic Medicine: The Principles of Traditional Practice. Churchill Livingston Elsevier, 2006; 296-297.

67 Inaba, R., Mirbod, S.M, and Sugiura, H. Effects of maharishi amrit kalash 5 as an Ayurvedic herbal food supplement on immune functions of aged mice. BMC Complement Altern Med. 2005; 5: 8.

68 Penza, M., et al. MAK-4 and -5 supplemented diet inhibits liver carcinogenesis in mice. BMC Complement Altern Med. 2007; 7-19.

69 Inaba, R., Sugiura, H., and Iwata, H. Immunomodulatory effects of Maharishi Amrit Kalash 4 and 5 in mice. Nihon Eiseigaku Zasshi. 1995; 50(4): 901-5.

70 Vohra, B.P., Sharma, S.P., Kansai, V.K. Maharishi Amrit Kalash rejuvenates ageing central nervous system's antioxidant defense system: an in vivo study. Pharmacol Res. 1999; 40(6): 497-502.

71   Lenzi, M., Fimognari, C., and Hrelia P. Sulforaphane as a promising molecule for fighting cancer. Adv Nutr Cancer. 2013; 159: 207-23.

72   Kumar, S. and Pandey, A.K. Chemistry and biological activities of flavonoids: an overview. Scientific World Journal. 2013; 162750.

73   Zhu, X., et al. Polyphenol extract of Phyllanthus emblica (PEEP) induces inhibition of cell proliferation and triggers apoptosis in cervical cancer cells. 2013; 18(1): 46.

74   De, A., et al. Emblica officinalis extract induces autophagy and inhibits human ovarian cancer cell proliferation, angiogenesis, growth of mouse xenograft tumors. PLoS One. 2013; 8(8): e72748.

75   Poltanov, E.A., et al. Chemical and antioxidant evaluation of Indian gooseberry supplements. Phytother Res. 2009; 23(9): 1309-15.

76   Deb, A., Barua, S., and Das, B. Pharmacological activities of Baheda (Terminalia bellerica): A review. J Pharmacog and Phytochem. 2016; 5(1): 194-7.

77   Usharani, P., et al. A randomized, double-blind, placebo, and positive-controlled clinical pilot study to evaluate the efficacy and tolerability of standardized aqueous extracts of Terminalia chebula and Terminalia bellerica in subjects with hyperuricemia.

78   Lee, M.S., et al. Maca (Lepidium meyenii) for treatment of menopausal symptoms: A systematic review. Maturitas. 2011; 70(3): 227-33.

79   Stone, M., et al. A pilot investigation into the effect of maca supplementation on physical activity and sexual desire in sportsmen. J Ethnopharmacol. 2009; 126(3): 574-6.

80   Gonzales, G.F., et al. Effect of Lepidium meyenii (MACA) on sexual desire and its relationship with serum testosterone levels in adult healthy men. Andrologia. 2002; 34(6): 367-72.

81   Shin, B.C., et al. Maca (L. meyenii) for improving sexual function: a systematic review. BMC Complement Altern Med. 2010; 10: 44.

82   Brooks, N.A., et al. Beneficial effects of Lepidium meyenii (Maca) on psychological symptoms and measures of sexual dysfunction in

postmenopausal women are not related to estrogen or androgen content. Menopause. 2008; 15(6): 1157-62.

83 Stojanovska, L. et al. Maca reduces blood pressure and depression, in a pilot study in postmenopausal women. Climacteric. 2015; 18(1): 69-78.

84 Guo, S.S., et al. Preservation of cognitive function by Lepidium meyenii (Maca) is associated with improvement of mitochondrial activity and upregulation of autophagy-related proteins in middle-aged mouse cortex. Evid Based Complement Alternat Med. 2016; 4394261. Epub.

85 Weiss, D.J. and Anderton, C.R. Determination of catechins in matcha green tea by micellar electrokinetic chromatography. J Chromatogr A. 2003; 11(1-2): 173-80.

86 Pham-Huy, L.A., He, H., and Pham-Huy, C. Free radicals, antioxidants in disease and health. Int J Biomed Sci. 2008; 4(2): 89-96.

87 Dietz, C., Dekker, M., and Piqueras-Fiszman, B. An intervention study on the effect of matcha tea, in drink and snack bar formats, on mood and cognitive performance. Food Res Int. 2017; 99(pt 1): 72-83.

88 Nobre, A.C., Rao, A., and Owen, G.N. L-theanine, a natural tea constituent in tea, and its effect on mental state. Asia Pac J Clin Nutr. 2008; 1: 167-8.

89 Kavanagh, K.T., et al. Green tea extracts decrease carcinogen-induced mammary tumor burden in rats and rate of breast cancer cell proliferation in culture. J Cell Biochem. 2001; 82(3): 387-98.

90 University of Michigan Health System. Green tea compound, ECGC, may be therapy for people with rheumatoid arthritis. Science Daily. 2007. www.sciencedaily.com/releases/2007/04/070429113444.htm

91 Boyle, N.B., Lawton, C., and Dye, L. The effects of magnesium supplementation on subjective anxiety and stress – A systematic review. Nutrients. 2017; 9(5): 429.

92 Tassabehji, N.M., et al. Zinc deficiency induces depression-like symptoms in adult rats. Physiol Behav. 2008; 95(3): 365-9.

93 Whittle, N., Lubec, G., and Singewald, N. Zinc deficiency induces enhanced depression-like behavior and altered limbic activation

reversed by antidepressant treatment in mice. Amino Acids. 2009; 36(1): 147-58.

94 Cope, E.C. and Levenson, C.W. Role of zinc in the development and treatment of mood disorders. Curr Opin Clin Nutr Metab Care. 2010; 13(6): 685-9.

95 Xu, Y., et al. Novel therapeutic targets in depression and anxiety: antioxidants as candidate treatment. Curr Neuropharmacol. 2014; 12(2): 108-19.

96 Ashley-Farrand, T. Mantra: Sacred Words of Power. Study Guide. Sounds True. 1999; pp. 23-24.

97 Ibid, pp. 24.

98 Yackle, K., et al. Breathing control center neurons that promote arousal in mice. Science. 2017; 355(6332): 1411-15.

99 Szewczyk, B., Kotarska, K., Daigle, M., Misztak, P., Sowa-Kucma, M., Rafalo, A., Curzytek, K., Kubera, M., Basta-Kaim, A., Nowak, G., Albert, P.R. Stress-induced alterations in 5-HT1A receptor transcriptional modulators NUDR and Freud-1. Int J Neuropsychopharmacol. 2014; Jun 19:1-13. Epub.

100 Karssen, A.M., Her S, Li, J.Z., Patel, P.D., Meng, F., Bunney, W.E. Jr, Jones, E.G., Watson, S.J., Akil, H., Myers, R.M., Schatzberg, A.F., Lyons, D.M. Stress-induced changes in primate prefrontal profiles of gene expression. Mol Psychiatry. 2007; 12(12):1089-102.

101 Kant G.J., et al. Effects of controllable vs. uncontrollable chronic stress-responsive plasma hormones. Physiol Behav. 1992; 51(6): 1285-8.

102 Garbett, K.A., Vereczkei, A., Kálmán, S., Brown, J.A., Taylor, W.D., Faludi, G., Korade, Z., Shelton, R.C., Mirnics, K. Coordinated Messenger RNA/MicroRNA Changes in Fibroblasts of Patients with Major Depression. Biol Psychiatry. 2014; Jun 2. pii: S0006-3223(14)00376-X. doi: 10.1016/j.biopsych.2014.05.015. [Epub

103 Nishi, M., Horii-Hayashi, N., Sasagawa, T. Effects of early life adverse experiences on the brain: implications from maternal sepa-

ration models in rodents. Front Neurosci. 2014; Jun 17;8:166. doi: 10.3389/fnins.2014.00166. eCollection 2014. Review.

104 Ghetti, C.M. Active music engagement with emotional-approach coping to improve well-being in liver and kidney transplant recipients. J Music Ther. 2011; Winter;48(4):463-85.

105 Marchant, J. Immunology: The pursuit of happiness. Nature. 2013; Nov 28;503(7477):458-60. doi: 10.1038/503458a.

106 Powell, N.D., Sloan, E.K., Bailey, M.T., Arevalo, J.M., Miller, G.E., Chen, E., Kobor, M.S., Reader, B.F., Sheridan, J.F., Cole, S.W. Social stress up-regulates inflammatory gene expression in the leukocyte transcriptome via β-adrenergic induction of myelopoiesis. Proc Natl Acad Sci USA. 110(41):16574-9. doi: 10.1073/pnas.1310655110. Epub 2013 Sep 23.

107 Cole, S.W., Conti, G., Arevalo, J.M., Ruggiero, A.M., Heckman, J.J., Suomi, S.J. Transcriptional modulation of the developing immune system by early life social adversity. Proc Natl Acad Sci USA; 109(50):20578-83. doi: 10.1073/pnas.1218253109. Epub 2012 Nov 26.

108 Byrnes D.M., et al. Stressful events, pessimism, natural killer cell cytotoxicity, and cytotoxic/suppressor T cells in HIV+ black women at risk for cervical cancer. Psychomatic Med. 1998; 60(6): 714-22.

109 Hoffman, J.W., et al. Reduced sympathetic nervous system responsivity associated with the relaxation response. Science. 1982; 190-192.

110 https://www.thecrimson.com/article/1982/1/13/new-harvard-research-tells-how-meditation/

111 Bhasin, M.K. et al. Relaxation response induces temporal transcriptome changes in energy metabolism, insulin secretion and inflammatory pathways. PLoS ONE. 8(5): e62817.doi: 10.1371/journal.pone.0062871PMID: 23650531.

112 Stahl, J.E., et al. Relaxation response and resiliency training and its effects on healthcare resource utilization. PLoS ONE. 2015: https://doi.org/10.1371/journal.pone.0140212.

113 Krishnakumar D., Hamblin, M.R., and Lakshmanan, S. Meditation and yoga can modulate brain mechanisms that affect behavior and anxiety: A modern scientific perspective. Anc Sci. 2015; 2(1): 13-19.

114 Lang A.J., et al. The theoretical and empirical basis for meditation as an intervention for PTSD. Behavior Modification. 2012; 0145445512441200.

115 There is no particular reason for starting with the left foot. I do, however, often start with the left hand or foot.

116 In yoga, it is discussed in terms of subtle energy channels (ida, pingala, and sushumna nadis). To maintain energy balance, the flow of energy must be even and free through each of these channels. The ida swara is cooling, relaxing, and calming, and is associated with the feminine and lunar qualities; it terminates in the left nostril. The pingala swara is the solar channel associated masculine qualities and increases heat in the body along with energy and activity; it terminates in the right nostril.

117 Advanced students can also practice sahita kumbhaka, not described in this book, with or without mantra or affirmation.

118 Bhavanani, A.B., et al. Differential effects of uninostril and alternate nostril pranayamas on cardiovascular parameters and reaction time. Int J Yoga. 2014; 7(1): 60-5.

119 Raghuraj, P. and Telles, S. Immediate effect of specific nostril manipulating yoga breathing practices on autonomic and respiratory variables. Appl Psychophysiol Biofeedback. 2008; 33(2): 65-75.

120 Upadhyay, D.K., et al. Effect of alternate nostril breathing exercise on cardiorespiratory functions. Nepal Med Coll J. 2008; 10(1): 25-7.

121 Srivastava, R.D., Jain, N., and Singhal, A. Influence of alternate nostril breathing on cardiorespiratory and autonomic functions in healthy young adults. Indian J Physiol Pharmacol. 2005; 49(4): 475-83.

122 Field, T., et al. Cortisol decreases and serotonin and dopamine increase following massage therapy. Int J Neruosci. 2005; 115(10): 1397-413.

123 The oil type varies with body type, which is determined by an experienced Ayurvedic physician or health counselor. Vatas benefit the most from sesame oil, pittas from sunflower or coconut, and kaphas from corn oil.

124 Alexander, C.N., Rainforth, M.V., and Gelderloos, P. Transcendental meditation, self-actualization, and psychological health: a conceptual overview and statistical meta-analysis. J Social Behavior and Personality. 1991; 6(5): 189-247.

125 Chandler, H.M., Alexander, C.M., and Heaton, D.P. The Transcendental Meditation program and postconventional self-development: a 10-year longitudinal study. Consciousness-Based Education. 2011; 2: 382-419.

126 Sherman, G.D., et al. Leadership is associated with lower levels of stress. Proc Natl Acad Sci. 2012; www.pnas.org/doi/10.1073/pnas.1207042109.

127 Guyon, A., et al. Adverse effects of two nights of sleep restriction on the hypothalamic-pituitary-adrenal axis in healthy men. J Clin Endocrinol Metab. 2014; 99(8): 2861-8.

128 Minkel, J., et al. Sleep deprivation potentiates HPA axis stress reactivity in healthy adults. Health Psychol. 2014; 33(11): 1430-4.

129 Vgontzas, A., et al. Chronic insomnia is associated with nyctohemeral activation of the hypothalamic-pituitary-adrenal axis: clinical implications. J Clin Endocrinol Metab. 2001; 86: 3787-94.

130 Bierwolf, C., et al. Slow wave sleep drives inhibition of pituitary-adrenal secretion in humans. J Neuroendocrinol. 1997; 9: 479-84.

131 Weitzman, E.D., et al. Cortisol secretion is inhibited during sleep in normal man. J Clin Endocrinol Metab. 1983; 56: 352-58.

132 Spath-Schwalbe, E., et al. Corticotropin-releasing hormone-induced adrenocorticotropin and cortisol secretion depends on sleep and wakefulness. J Clin Endocrinol Metab. 1993; 77: 1170-73.

133 Bush, B. and Hudson, T. The role of Cortisol in Sleep. Natural Med J. 2010 2(6): https://www.naturalmedicinejournal.com/journal/2010-06/role-cortisol-sleep.

134 Vgontzas, A., et al. Chronic insomnia and the activity of the stress system: a preliminary study. J Psychosom Res. 1998. 45: 21-31.

135 Rodenback, A., et al. Interactions between evening and nocturnal cortisol secretion and sleep parameters in patients with severe chronic primary insomnia. Neurosci Lett. 2002; 324: 159-163.

136 Meerlo, P., Sgoifo, A. and Suchecki, D. Restricted and disrupted sleep: Effects on autonomic function, neuroendocrine stress systems, and stress responsivity. Sleep Med Rev. 2008; 12: 197-210.

137 Dahlgren, A., Kecklund, G., and Akerstedt, T. Different levels of work-related stress and the effects on sleep, fatigue, and cortisol. Scand J Work Environ Heatlh. 2005; 31(4): 277-285.

138 McEwen, B.S. Stressed or stressed out: What is the difference? J Psychiatry Neurosci. 2005; 30(5): 315-318.

139 Juster, R-P., McEwen, B.S. Sleep and chronic stress: new directions for allostatic load research. Sleep Med. 2015; 16(1): 7-8.

140 Rinse with saline solution (half a teaspoon to begin with and increase to one teaspoon). Use room temperature to lukewarm water. Repeated use may dry out the nasal passage; therefore, apply some warm sesame oil to the entrance of the nostril with a cotton swab as needed. After rinsing sinuses, practice Kapalabhati (bellows breath) by inhaling and sharply contracting your lower abdomen to expel air vigorously. Do this rapidly (ten to twenty times) and keep accentuating the exhale with your abdomen and intercostal muscles. You can do a standing forward bend to let your sinuses drain afterwards, as well. This process is called Neti Kriya.

141 Jacobs, G.D., Benson, H., and Friedman, R. Perceived benefits in a behavioral-medicine insomnia program: a clinical report. AmJ Med. 1996; 100(2): 212-6.

142 Cole, R.J. Postural baroreflex stimuli may affect EEG arousal and sleep in humans. J Appl Physiol. 1989; 67(6): 2369-75.

143 Shannahoff-Khalsa, D.S. Kundalini Yoga Meditation: Techniques Specific for Psychiatric Disorders, Couples Therapy & Personal Growth. W.W. Norton. 2006; pp. 170-172.

144 Shannahoff-Khalsa, D.S An introduction to Kundalini yoga meditation techniques that are specific for the treatment of psychiatric disorders. J Altern Complement Med. 2004; 10(1): 91-101.

145 Swami Veda Bharati. My experiments with yoga nidra. Himalayan Publications Trust. Amazon Digital Services LLC. 2015.

146 Patak, P. Willenberg, H., and Bornstein, S. Vitamin C is an important co-factor for both adrenal cortex and adrenal medulla. Endoc Res. 2004; 30: 871-5.

147 Srivastava, J.K., Shankar, E., and Gupta, S. Chamomile: A herbal medicine of the past with bright future. Mol Med Report. 2010; 3(6): 895-901.

148 Howatson, G., et al. Effect of tart cherry juice (Prunus cerasus) on melatonin levels and enhanced sleep quality. Eur J Nutr. 2012; 51(8): 909-16.

149 Melatonin is a hormone made by the pineal gland that regulates sleep/wake cycles. Secretion increases in darkness or at night. Melatonin (1-3 mg ideally) can be taken two hours before bedtime. If it does not help after a couple of weeks, discontinue its use. Typically, it is safe to take for 1-2 months. However, finding a more permanent and internal option, like I discuss in this book, would be the best option.

150 Grandner, M.A., et al. Dietary nutrients associated with short and long sleep duration. Data from a nationally representative sample. Appetite. 2013; 64: 71-80.

151 Lad, V. The complete book of ayurvedic home remedies. Three Rivers Press. 1998; pp. 211-212.

152 Snell, P. Women's stress upped by irregular work schedules. 2004; http://womenof.com, Prosolutions, Inc.

153 Paramahansa Yogananda. Scientific Healing Affirmations: Theory and Practice of Concentration. Self-Realization Fellowship, 2007.

154 The Five Yamas are: (1) Ahimsa or non-violence, (2) Satya or truthfulness, (3) Asteya or non-stealing, (4) Bramacharya or non-excess, and (5) aparigraha or non-possesiveness.

The Five Niyamas are: (1) saucha or purity, (2) santosha or contentment, (3) tapas or self-discipline, (4) svadhyaya or inner self-study, and (5) ishvara pranidhana or self-surrender.

155 Identify what events activate your monkey mind more. How are you interpreting these events in your mind? Are you judging, imprinting your beliefs or preconceptions? What are the consequences of your thoughts? How do you feel afterwards?

156 Frawley, D. Ayurveda and the mind: The healing of consciousness. Lotus Press. 1996; pp. 175.

157 Stimulation with the right sensory impressions varies depending on your predominant dosha, or the energy makeup that defines you. For a description, please refer to: Frawley, D. Ayurveda and the mind: The healing of consciousness. Lotus Press.1996; pp. 183-186.

158 Maddi, S.R. Hardiness: Turning stressful circumstances into resilient growth. Springer. 2013.

159 Ashley-Farrand, T. Healing mantras: Using sound affirmations for personal power, health, and creativity. Sounds True. 1999; pp. 7-8.

160 Ibid, pp. 15.

161 Kaur, S. Meditation of the Soul: 11 Recitations of the Pauris of Jap Ji. Spirit Voyage. 2015.

162 Shannahoff-Khalsa, D.S. Kundalini Yoga Meditation: Techniques Specific for Psychiatric Disorders, Couples Therapy & Personal Growth. W.W. Norton. 2006; pp. 79.

163 Shih, C.M., et al. Anti-inflammatory and antihyperalgesic activity of C-phycocyanin. Anesth Analg. 2009; 108(4): 1303-10.

164 Farooq, S.M., et al. C-phycocyanin confers protection against oxalate-mediated oxidative stress and mitochondrial dysfunctions in MDCK cells. PLoS One. 2014; 9(4): e93056.

165 Romay, C.H. C-phycocyanin: a biliprotein with antioxidant, anti-inflammatory, and neuroprotective effects. Curr Protein Pept Sci. 2003; 4(3): 207-16.

166 Ismail, M.F., et al. Chemoprevention of rat liver toxicity and carcinogenesis by Spirulina. Int J Biol Sci. 2009; 5(4): 377-87.

167 Akao, Y., et al. Enhancement of antitumor natural killer cell activation by orally administered Spirulina extract in mice. Cancer Sci. 2009; 100(8): 1494-501.

168 Mathew, B., et al. Evaluation of chemoprevention of oral cancer with Spirulina fusiformis. Nutr Cancer. 1995; 24(2): 197-202.

169 Kalafati, M., et al. Ergogenic and antioxidant effects of spirulina supplementation in humans. Med Sci Sports Exerc. 2010; 42(1): 142-51.

170 Queiroz, M.L., et al. Protective Effects of Chlorella vulgaris in lead-exposed mice infected with Listeria monocytogenes. Int Immunopharmacol. 2003; 3(6): 889-900.

171 Uchikawa, T., et al. Enhanced elimination of tissue methylmercury in Parachlorella beijerinckii-fed mice. J Toxicol Sci. 2011; 36(1): 121-6.

172 Otsuki, T., et al. Salivary secretory immunoglobulin A secretion increases after 4-weeks ingestion of chlorella-derived multicomponent supplement in humans: a randomized cross over study. Nutr J. 2011; 10: 91.

173 Kwak, J.H., et al. Beneficial immunostimulatory effect of short-term Chlorella supplementation: enhancement of natural killer cell activity and early inflammation response (randomized, double-blinded, placebo-controlled trial). Nutr J. 2012; 11: 53.

174 Lordan, S., Ross, R., and Stanton, C. Marine bioactives as functional food ingredients: Potential to reduce the incidence of chronic diseases. Mar Drugs. 2011; 9(6): 1056-1100.

175 Makpol, S., et al. Chlorella vulgaris modulates hydrogen peroxide-induced DNA damage and telomere shortening of human fibroblasts derived from different aged individuals. Afr J Tradit Complement Altern Med. 2009; 6(4): 560-72.

176 Hillmire, M.R., DeVylder, J.E., and Forestell, C.A. Fermented foods, neuroticism, and social anxiety: an interaction model. Psychiatry Res. 2015; 228(2): 203-8.

177 Park, E.Y., et al. Efficacy comparisons of Korean ginseng and American ginseng on body temperature and metabolic parameters. Am J Chin Med. 2014; 42(1): 173-87.

178 Kim, D.H. Chemical diversity of panax ginseng, panax quinquifolium, and panax notoginseng. J Ginseng Res. 2012; 36(1): 1-15.

179 Park, B.G., et al. Potentiation of antioxidative and anti-inflammatory properties of cultured wild ginseng root extract through probiotic fermentation. J Pharm Pharmacol. 2013; 65(3): 457-64.

180 Scholey, A., et al. Effect of American ginseng (Panax quinquefolius) on neurocognitive function: an acute, randomized, double-blind, placebo-controlled, crossover study. Psychopharm. 2010; 212(3): 345-356.

181 Inoue, T., et al. Tropical fruit camu-camu (Myrciaria dubia) has anti-oxidative and anti-inflammatory properties. J Cardiol. 2008; 52(2): 127-32.

182 Howitz, K.T., et al. Small molecule activators of sirtuins extend Saccharomyces cerevisiae lifespan. Nature. 2003; 425(6954): 191-6.

183 Granzotto A. and Zatta, P. Resveratrol and Alzheimer's disease: message in a bottle on red wine and cognition. Front Aging Neurosci. 2014; 6: 95.

184 Braidy, N., et al. Resveratrol as a potential therapeutic candidate for the treatment and management of Alzheimer's disease. Curr Top Med Chem. 2016; 16(17): 1951-60.

185 Moussa, C., et al. Resveratrol regulates neuro-inflammation and induces adaptive immunity in Alzheimer's disease. J Neuroinflammation. 2017; 14(1): 1.

186 Zulueta, A., et al. Resveratrol: A potential challenger against gastric cancer. World J Gastroenterol. 2015; 21(37): 10636-43.

187 Tessitore, L., et al. Resveratrol depresses the growth of colorectal aberrant crypt foci by affecting bax and p21 (CIP) expression. Carcinogenesis. 2000; 21(8): 1619-22.

188 Raudenbush, B., et al. Effects of peppermint and cinnamon odor administration on simulated driving alertness, mood, and workload. N Am J Psychol. 2009; 11(2): 245-56.

189 Nehlig, A. The neuroprotective effects of cocoa flavonol and its influence on cognitive performance. Br J Clin Pharmacol. 2013; 75(3): 716-27.

190 Sorond, F.A., et al. Cerebral blood flow response to flavanol-rich cocoa in healthy elderly humans. Neuropsychiatr Dis Treat. 2008; 4(2): 433-40.

191 Araujo, Q.R., et al. Cocoa and human health: From head to foot—A review. Crit Rev Food Sci Nutr. 2016; 56(1): 1-12.

192 Ried, K., Fakler, P., and Stocks, N.P. Effect of cocoa on blood pressure. Cochrane Database Syst Rev. 2017; 4: CD008893.

193 Sokolov, A.N., et al. Chocolate and the brain: neurobiological impact of cocoa flavanols on cognition and behavior. Neurosci Biobehav Rev. 2013; 37(10 Pt 2): 2445-53.

194 Strandberg, T.E., et al. Chocolate, well-being and health among elderly men. Eur J Clin Nutr. 2008; 62(2): 247-53.

195 Balint, G., et al. Effect of Avemar—a fermented wheat germ extract—on rheumatoid arthritis. Preliminary data. Clin Exp Rheumatol. 2006; 24(3): 325-8.

196 Telekes, A., et al. Fermented wheat germ extract (avemar) inhibits adjuvant arthritis. Ann NY Acad Sci. 2007; 1110: 348-61.

197 Lake, J. H. and Spiegel, D. Complementary and Alternative Treatments in Mental Health Care. Ch 7: Omega-3 Essential Fatty Acids. American Psychiatric Publishing. 2007; pp. 151-67.

198 Consult your physician before taking, especially if taking certain medications.

199 Genaro, K., et al. Cannabidiol is a potential therapeutic for the affective-motivational dimension of incision pain in rats. Front Pharmacol. 2017; 8: 391.

200 Costa, B., et al. The non-psychoactive cannabis constituent cannabidiol is an orally effective therapeutic agent in rat chronic inflammatory and neuropathic pain. Eur J Pharmacol. 2007; 556(1-3): 75-83.

201 Hay, G.L, et al. Cannabidiol treatment reduces the motivation to self-administer methamphetamine and methamphetamine-primed relapse in rats. J Psychopharm. 2018; 32(12): 1277-85.

202 Bergamaschi, M.M., et al. Cannabidiol reduces the anxiety induced by simulated public speaking in treatment-naïve social phobia patients. Neuropsychopharmacol. 2011; 36(6): 1219-26.

203 Shannon, S. Effectiveness of cannabidiol oil for pediatric anxiety and insomnia as part of posttraumatic stress disorder: A case report. Perm J. 2016; 20(4): 108-111.

204 Blessing, E.M., et al. Cannabidiol as a potential treatment for anxiety disorders. Neurotherapeutics. 2015; 12(4): 825-36.

205 Jadoon, K.A., Tan, G.D., and O'Sullivan, S.E. A single dose of cannabidiol reduces blood pressure in healthy volunteers in a randomized crossover study. JCL Insight. 2017; 2(12): e93760.

206 Whitehead, A., et al. Cholesterol-lowering effects of oat beta-glucan: a meta-analysis of randomized controlled trials. Am J Clin Nutr. 2014; 100(6): 1413-21.

207 Chen, J. and Raymond, K. Beta-glucan in the treatment of diabetes and associated cardiovascular risks. Vasc Health Risk Manag. 2008; 4(6): 1265-72.

208 El Khoury, D., et al. Beta-glucan: health benefits in obesity and metabolic syndrome. J Nutr Metab. 2012; 851362. Epub.

209 Sohrab, G., et al. Effects of pomegranate juice consumption on inflammatory markers in patients with type-2 diabetes: A randomized, placebo-controlled trial. J Res Med Sci. 2014; 19(3): 215-20.

210 Pantuck, A.J., et al. Phase II study of pomegranate juice for men with rising prostate-specific antigen following surgery or radiation for prostate cancer. Clin Cancer Res. 2006; 12(13): 4018-26.

211 Hartman, R.E., et al. Pomegranate juice decreases amyloid load and improves behavior in a mouse model of Alzheimer's disease. Neurobiol Dis. 2006; 24(3): 506-15.

212 Amagase, H. and Nance, D.M. A randomized, double-blind, placebo-controlled, clinical study of the general effects of a standardized Lycium barbarum (goji) Juice, GoChi. J Altern Complement Med. 2008; 14(4): 403-12.

9 781642 795806